SACRED BALANCE

SACRED BALANCE

Aligning Body and Spirit through Yoga and the Benedictine Way

Illustrations: Gisela Bohórquez
Cover design: James Kegley

Print ISBN: 978-1-5064-6353-7
eBook ISBN: 978-1-5064-6354-4

SACRED BALANCE

ALIGNING BODY AND SPIRIT THROUGH
YOGA AND THE BENEDICTINE WAY

MELINDA EMILY THOMAS

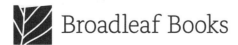 Broadleaf Books

For my Grandma Dorothy,
a woman of deep faith who was always there

CONTENTS

PREFACE

As the child of an Episcopal priest, I grew up in a world steeped in spirituality. Both of my parents studied, taught, and ministered in their own ways. Yet my introduction to the balancing tradition of the Rule of St. Benedict came not from my parents but from a collection of mystery novels on their bookshelves. Set on the Welsh–English border, the Chronicles of Brother Cadfael, a mystery series written by Edith Mary Pargeter under the pen name Ellis Peters, revolves around Brother Cadfael, a fictional twelfth-century crusader turned Benedictine monk, herbalist, and solver of murders. The series is filled with theology, compassion, and grace. The ill, the rich, the poor, the stranger, the friend, the criminal, the refugee, and the citizen all received hospitality at the monastery table, which stands at the heart of Benedictine tradition. In the wandering, interior days of a severe depression I experienced during college, Cadfael's abbey became my sanctuary and offered a new way to understand how values and spirituality could be combined in a profound set of practices.

That depression was not my first episode of mental illness, nor would it be my last. Oscillating between bouts of depression, anxiety, excitability, evenness, physical pain, and chronic fatigue, I spent my twenties and early-to mid-thirties out of balance. That difficult period became the catalyst and proving ground for my inner and outer orientation toward sacred balance.

As a teenager I was drawn to the practice of yoga as an expression of spirit. During the height of my illness, I felt a deep yearning and affinity toward yoga and knew it was where God was calling me to be. After taking a few classes at local yoga studios, I found a teacher with whom I resonated and began an intensive period of study. Even when I couldn't be active for more than a few hours a day, I could practice yoga. When my moods became debilitating, I could practice yoga. In the marriage of breath and posture, in the study of philosophy and meditation, in the discipline of daily practice, in the support of community, I found healing and balance.

In this journey I have come to learn that balance is not static. Balance is a dynamic response to the ever-shifting currents of life. Maintaining balance is not a matter of hardening the body or spirit. Rather, it is a matter of steady muscular engagement and internal focus that allows for the natural contraction and expansion of muscles and breath. It's much like standing on one leg in some yoga poses: When I brace against the subtle movement of the standing foot, I fall. When I don't engage enough focused physical and mental energy paired with fluid breath, I fall. Balance is the conversation that happens between steadiness and movement.

Because balance is a dynamic response rather than an elusive goal, *Sacred Balance* is built on reflection and practice. This book is a conversation between the two primary structures that bring balance to my life: Benedictine spirituality and yoga.

The simple yet profound principles of the Way of St. Benedict will be infused with the life-giving practices of yoga and *Ayurveda*. Ayurveda, the sister science of yoga, draws its wisdom from the observation of how nature keeps itself in balance. The berries of summer cool the season's heat. Cinnamon and cardamom warm the body in winter. Quiet breathing steadies an overactive mind. Well-being is found in the interplay of opposites working together to find harmony.

The gentle, uncomplicated practices of Ayurveda offered in this book are not intended to diagnose or treat any medical disease. They are intended to enhance wellness and perhaps bring a new perspective on balance. As with any health regime, it is always best to consult with a licensed professional.

A good, working principle that has guided me along this path is asking two questions that help locate imbalance:

- Am I honestly living the practices that care for my physical and spiritual well-being?
- Am I doing the things that I know bring a sense of equanimity and fulfillment in my life?

There are several answers you might come to. One may be yes, you are caring for yourself through practices such as journaling, prayer, reaching out to friends, eating well, getting outside, and spending time in ways that are meaningful to you. Or perhaps your old ways of finding balance no longer feel nourishing and it is time to make a change, to let some practices go or to explore new ones. Perhaps you are nurturing your body, mind, and spirit but you still feel out of balance. That may be the time to seek additional guidance, whether from a friend, a teacher, a spiritual director, or a professional clinician.

The path of balance is simple in its poetry because it embraces what is beautiful and life-giving. Benedictine spirituality and yoga affirm what is holy about who we are and give us tangible means to explore the harmony of mind, body, and heart.

As Benedict writes in the opening lines of his sixth-century Rule for monastics, "Listen carefully, my child, to my instructions, and attend to them with the ear of your heart. This is advice from one who loves you; welcome it and faithfully put it into practice."

I share with you the practices passed on to me from many teachers, spiritual guides, and loved ones. May they inspire you on this path of sacred balance.

HOW TO USE THIS BOOK

Benedictine spirituality and yoga are more than just philosophies to be studied; they are practices to be lived. The yogis and yoginis (practitioners of yoga, male and female) have a word for this: *abhyasa*, or "steady effort over time." To foster that balance, this book is practice-focused. Each chapter begins with a reflection on a Benedictine principle and its yogic complement, considering how they relate to the path of balance. A series of gentle, easy-to-implement exercises comes next. These will include questions for reflection, a wellness practice, a prayer or meditation, and a short sequence of yoga postures that embody the theme of the chapter. Each yoga pose, also called an *asana*, is accompanied by an illustration and notes on modifications. Modifications not pictured in the book can be found on my website, www.TheHouseholdersPath.com.

Props that will aid your practice include:

- yoga mat
- two blocks
- two or three blankets
- a small dish or hand towel
- bolster (optional)

You can use blankets from around your house. I encourage you to invest in a yoga mat and blocks, as they are valuable additions for your practice. These tools can be purchased at just about any sporting goods or health food store, as well as at most major retailers and online vendors. A bolster is a bonus but not necessary—blankets can be used in its place.

I encourage you to read through each asana sequence in full. While many of the poses are repeated, I offer guidance on how to approach the posture from an inward focus that matches the theme of the chapter.

Some of the terms used in this work will be presented in Latin (the language of Benedict), some will be given in Sanskrit (the language of yoga), and at times I will include their English translations. I use these words to give you a new language with which to discuss balance. In doing so, you may be able to claim interior space that you haven't previously explored. A glossary of these terms is included in the back of the book. For the sake of simplicity, I have also removed the diacriticals (accents or notations that indicate a variation on pronounciation) on many of the Sanskrit words.

In addition, I will use multiple forms of language for God. God, Ground of Being, Self, Presence, Divine, Grace, Higher Power, Christ: in this book they all point to the sacred. I intentionally use a variety of terms in the hopes of offering a rich and accessible way for readers of all faiths or no faith to encounter holiness and to fold it into the path of sacred balance.

1

Stepping onto the Path of Balance

The spiritual life is a grace with which we must cooperate.

—Joan Chittister, OSB

In the earliest days of grade school we learn our primary colors: red, yellow, blue. Then the secondary colors: green, violet, orange. Next we learn that the primary and secondary colors complement each other: red and green, yellow and violet, blue and orange. Placed next to each other, complementary colors each enhance the other's hue, creating a sense of equanimity. Color is waves of light. Modern physics has shown that light is both a particle and a wave— steadiness and movement. The equanimity we feel when complementary colors are next to each other is the resonance of particles and waves in harmonious action.

We often envision balance in terms of a balance-beam scale—one of those old scales with the single horizontal beam from which two trays hang. When the objects in each tray are of equal weight, the scale is in balance. While this may be true for purposes of measurement, it is unhelpful and perhaps even harmful to think of balanced living in terms of a scale. When we conceptualize balance in this way, we risk stasis and perfectionism. Life is not static. We are always growing and changing in response to circumstances and relationships. Perfection is an insidious and unattainable goal, defined by subjective externals, rather than an enthusiastic exploration of the fullness of our humanity.

Instead, I prefer to think of balance in terms of color theory. Harmony and well-being are found when the particles and waves—the steadiness *and* the motion—of our lives amplify or counteract each other. Balanced living is not found in the mere elimination of one color or the addition of another. Balanced living is found in the conversation between the colors that are already there. It is the dialogue that matters.

When we feel overexcited, overworked, worn down, or depleted, we know something is out of whack. Some part of our daily routine is dominating the conversation. All too often the stresses of life—the demands of work and family, the bombardment of media, the countless messages about being more successful or productive—drown out the quieting voice of the heart longing to be heard. Sacred balance is restored through practices that promote an interior and exterior orientation toward God—the Ground of Being from which health and wellness spring. The interior orientation includes our priorities, attitudes, and values, which drive our external actions. Our external actions nurture and grow our healthy inner selves. We cannot have one without the other.

The mission of the YMCA, where I work as a coordinator of the Mind-Body program, is, "To put Christian principles into practice through programs that build healthy spirit, mind, and body for all." Spirit, mind, and body: our primary colors. For all: the rich diversity of every color in the spectrum, every part of our lives. Principles into practice: conversation with the colors of our days. Rooted in the Christian tradition, Benedictine spirituality is grounded in the understanding that God's presence is everywhere, in every color. While yoga, like Christianity, has many lineages, it too is anchored in the recognition that the Divine dwells within and without and that our path is to remember that wisdom.

I see Benedictine spirituality and yoga as complementary colors, each with its own hue and vibrance. My intent in this book is to illuminate how the two traditions enhance and mutually reinforce each other. I don't intend to paint them over each other and get a muddled mess; I intend to highlight the specifics of each as complementary.

Before we begin the dynamic conversation between the colors of Benedictine spirituality and yoga, it is helpful to have a general knowledge of the starting point for each tradition.

The Rule of St. Benedict

St. Benedict of Nursia was born in 480 CE in Umbria, Italy. The Roman Empire had fallen. Chaos, violence, and uncertainty filled the atmosphere of European life. The child of a relatively well-off family, Benedict was sent to Rome to study, but he left in favor of a contemplative life as a hermit in a hillside cave in Subiaco, east of Rome. His countercultural choice to live apart from society was likely not as rare as one might think. Monastics in the early sixth century included hermits, some communal orders, and wandering monks with no sense of place (or, as Benedict saw it, no spiritual purpose). Although he lived a solitary existence, he was eventually found by others, and within a few years he had started a small order of brothers, which eventually expanded to twelve small monasteries in the region. In the mid-520s Benedict and a few of his monks left Subiaco and established an order in the mountains of Monte Cassino, where he lived until his death in 540. Within two centuries, Benedictine monasteries grew from communities of about a dozen monks or nuns to cornerstones of medieval life. They became safe havens for travelers and beacons of learning, integral to church and secular society.

It is in the context of the tumultuous post-Roman world that Benedict wrote a manuscript that has come to be known as the *Rule of Saint Benedict*, or simply, the Rule. The Rule was a way to orient the days of the monks toward a balance between ordinary business—cooking, cleaning, eating, tending to the sick, teaching children, earning a living—and the deep yearning for life centered in prayer. Benedict was a layperson, not a priest. His concerns were practical, not dogmatic. Above all, Benedict sought to create an environment in which care of the soul and a communal life in Christ were priorities.

Firmly rooted in the Christian tradition, the Rule is a guidebook for living the transformative love of the gospel, which calls us to welcome and advocate for the poor, marginalized, and oppressed, remain steadfast in compassion, and trust in God's faithfulness. Yet the Rule transcends any particular religious ideology, and in doing so, becomes wisdom. The wisdom tradition, sometimes called the perennial tradition, is the common thread found in all the world's many religions. The wisdom tradition is concerned with the meaning of the sacred, the relationship of humans with one another and the Divine, inner transformation, and the fundamentals of joy.

The main principles infused in the Rule, which become the guideposts for Benedictine spirituality and our path of balance, are humility, obedience, stability, conversion, hospitality, daily and seasonal rhythms, silence, and sabbath. The chapters in this book follow these guideposts.

Humility is the starting point. Humility is a perpetual state of openness to learn and grow that comes from the understanding that we don't know everything and that we cannot and should not do everything. We are not alone. Humility is about being in right relationship with God, ourselves, and the world around us. While we are not responsible for the workings of the entire universe, our places of business, or even our families, we do contribute to the matrix of being. Having a mature knowledge of what is and what is not within our sphere of influence, while connecting with a Higher Power and community to guide us, is the essence of humility.

Obedience is one of three vows taken by Benedictine monks and oblates. (Monks and nuns, sometimes called monastics, are men and women who have taken vows to live within a religious order. Oblates are people who generally live in regular society but who have affiliated themselves in some way to a monastic community.) Evolving from the Latin root *oboedire*, which means "to listen," obedience is about call and response. In the monastery, obedience is about saying yes to the directions of other members of the community, in particular to the abbot or abbess, who serves as the authority figure in a monastic community. Going deeper, obedience is also the principle of listening deeply to God's call in our lives and responding accordingly. Benedict is clear that we cannot always know how we are being called; it is the community that helps us discern how we as individuals best serve Christ through being wholly ourselves.

Stability is the vow of staying put. Within the monastic context, stability is the vow to remain in the community no matter what. On an internal level, stability is the commitment to stick with our routines, new or old, that bring us balance. It is the ability to stay with our difficult emotions and circumstances because they help us grow. Like humility and obedience, stability is not a directive to accept the unacceptable. We are never called to acquiesce to circumstances or relationships of violence, abuse, or degradation. Rather, true stability is about remaining rooted in response to God's call instead of following the whims of the moment or avoiding discomfort.

Benedict is the master of paradox. Just when he calls for the steady movements of obedience and stability, he throws that steadiness into balance with motion. The third vow is conversion: a dedication to continual growth. In living the principle of conversion, we acknowledge our inevitable shortcomings and open ourselves to wonder, change, and rebirth.

Hospitality is another balancing principle central to Benedictine spirituality. At the monastery, all guests are welcome regardless of social status, age, race, gender, or economy. Guests are to be received with warmth and treated as family and embodiments of Christ. We are called to do the same for ourselves and others. We practice hospitality by giving room for all parts of ourselves to exist, especially the parts we find difficult. With loving attention, we give each emotion and character trait a seat at the table. We don't indulge the worst parts of ourselves, but we don't resist them either. Radical hospitality is an act of love for the people God created us to be. When we extend this welcome to ourselves, we are better able to extend it to others.

Benedict knew that spiritual formation happens within the context of daily living, is so he created a rhythm that allowed for focused prayer and reverent attention to the mundane. With times that varied according to the seasons of the year, monastic life revolved around the Divine Office: the call to communal prayer seven times a day. Time between prayer was given to reading or study, manual labor, eating and drinking, and rest. In giving due attention to all facets of human existence, Benedict recognizes God's presence everywhere. Utensils in the kitchen are treated with as much reverence as vessels on the altar. Rest is as important as work, and work is meaningful as prayer.

Silence is part of rest and a balancing principle of obedience. Monastics are to keep silence whenever possible so they can maintain focus on the sacred present. Time is set aside, particularly after Compline (the final communal prayer before bed), to be silent. In a world clamoring with noise, silence is vital. Silence, however, is not the absence of noise but a state of inner quiet in which the spirit, mind, and body can rest in Presence.

Finally we are invited to the practice of sabbath. In the Rule, Sundays are to be observed without manual labor and with more time given to rest, study, and communal prayer. Sabbath is an act of reminding ourselves that the world will go on without us and that we are encouraged to relish the wonderful gifts of life.

On the path of balance, we humbly accept that we need help; listen and locate the places of imbalance, and how God is calling us to shift; stick with the practices that keep us in balance whether they are old and comfortable or new and uncertain; are open to growth, looking and feeling foolish as we try new things; give a loving welcome to all parts of ourselves and one another; and create sustainable rhythms that allow for periods of prayer, work, eating, rest, silence, and sabbath.

Yoga

An influential yogi of the twentieth century, B. K. S. Iyengar, writes that yoga is an "art, a science, and a philosophy." The term yoga has both active and passive meanings, which broadly refer to actions of harnessing and union. Yoga is the practice of embracing complementary opposites—light and dark, steadiness and movement, masculine and feminine, self and Self—through recognizing their union in the Divine. It is both the means of unification and the unification itself. The process and the goal.

In the New Testament, St. Paul writes, "For just as the body is one and has many members, and all the members of the body, though many are one body, so it is with Christ" (1 Corinthians 12:12 NSRV). In a similar way, yoga invites the practitioner on a journey to see and celebrate difference within the revelation of universal oneness.

Yoga tradition, which dates back more than five thousand years, is rooted in the wisdom literature of the *Vedas*, the *Upanishads*, the *Bhagavad Gita*, and a sweeping array of other texts. The movement practices as we know them in the West today are a relatively new development in this ancient path, which is as complex and diverse as humanity itself in its points of view on life, culture, holiness, and practice. Compared to the *Rule of Saint Benedict*, which is a simple, short, singular text, yoga is immense. Encapsulating it in any one term, philosophy, religion, or ideology does a disservice to the tradition. Yet while the approach may be different from the Benedictine Way given their differing philosophical starting points, the goals of the two traditions run parallel: a life of integrity lived in communion with the Divine.

On our path of sacred balance, we will draw primarily on the eight-limbed path of yoga as outlined in the *Yoga Sutras of Patanjali*, as well the basics of its health care relative, Ayurveda.

The *Yoga Sutras of Patanjali* comprise 196 aphorisms on the purpose and practice of yoga. They are about 2,000 to 2,500 years old. Patanjali may have been one man or several writers, and much of what is known about the origin of the Sutras is myth. What we do have is an oral tradition written down as text. In this text, Patanjali delineates eight "limbs," or aspects, of yoga:

1. **Yamas:** Moral and ethical guidelines for behavior
   Ahimsa: Nonviolence or unwillingness to do harm
   Satya: Truth, honesty
   Asteya: Non-stealing
   Brahmacharya: Walking with God, moderation, temperance
   Aparigraha: Non-clinging, letting go

2. **Niyamas:** Observances for self-discipline and spiritual study
   Shauca: Purity, cleanliness outside and in
   Santosha: Contentment
   Tapas: Burning zeal in practice, desire to know more,
      willingness to grow
   Svadhyaya: Study of Self and scriptures
   Ishvara Pranidhana: Surrender to God

3. **Asana:** Physical practice designed to prepare the body for meditation

4. **Pranayama:** Breathwork

5. **Pratyahara:** Withdrawal of the senses

6. **Dharana:** Concentration

7. **Dhyana:** Meditation or contemplation

8. **Samadhi:** State of ecstasy, or merging with the highest form of the Self

Alongside the *Yoga Sutras of Patanjali*, I will also use a small portion of
the *Nārada Bhakti Sūtras*, an exquisite text on Divine Love and devotion (with
translation and commentary by yoga and Sanskrit scholar William K. Mahony,
PhD). I hope it enriches your path.

Much of the yoga that is practiced in Western society, with our focus on
movement and breathwork, is considered *hatha yoga*. In the same way that

Christianity has many denominations, hatha yoga has many lineages: Ashtanga, Iyengar, Anusara, Bikram, Vinyasa Flow, Jivamukti, and Yin are all examples of hatha yoga. Some lineages of hatha yoga are more gentle in their application of asanas than others.

Hatha yoga is a spiritual practice using primarily *asana* and *pranayama*—movement and breath—as the main tools. Yet to truly live a hatha yogic life, one must also incorporate the other six limbs of the eight-limbed path. Just as Benedict trusts that his monks will undertake the prayer and work of their days with the right attitude and actions arising from their longing for Christ, a yogi or yogini does so with the same emphasis of right attitude that underlies action both on and off the mat.

My approach to asana is born from the root intention of hatha yoga and is a primary component of my lived spirituality. Poses are practiced and experienced from the inside out. Each time I step onto my mat and attend to the movement of my body and breath, I create space for God's presence in my life. On the mat I practice being humble, steady, and easeful; listening; growing; welcoming being silent; and being at rest. The asana sequences in this book are offered with instruction on how to approach each pose from the inside out. The accompanying illustrations are included for further guidance. Additional modifications can be found on my website: www.TheHouseholdersPath.com. Many of the poses will be repeated, as the sequences build upon the foundation of those prior. I encourage you to read the instructions for each pose carefully. Although the basic alignment of poses may be the same across chapters, in each chapter I outline how to express the Benedictine and yogic principles we've looked at in that chapter within the pose.

Pranayama is also featured as a tool for balance. *Prana* is the yogic term for breath, life force, soul vitality. In Taoist tradition, it is called *chi*. In Hebrew, *ruach*. Christians might align the term with the Holy Spirit. Pranayamas are practices for rhythmic expansion or control of the breath that seek to harmonize and distribute the life-giving energy of prana throughout the body, mind, and spirit. The most basic pranayama is to train ourselves to allow the breath to lead the pose rather than to rely on willpower. We will focus on this throughout the asanas in this book. Chapter 8 will also include a specialized pranayama technique to give you another tool for balanced living.

Ayurveda

Ayurveda is a traditional health system for well-being. Often called the sister science to yoga, Ayurveda looks at patterns in the natural world to create blueprints for balanced living that can sometimes prevent or heal disease. While a sophisticated medical modality with a history of efficacy that spans millennia, Ayurveda also has a lovely simplicity that will guide our framework for balance. For our purposes, we will focus on the basic practices of *dina charya*—daily routines—and *ritu charya*—seasonal routines.

Central to Ayurveda is the concept of *doshas*. Doshas are forces of nature resulting from the interplay of the elements of space, earth, water, fire, and air, and are found in material and non material levels of existence. There are three doshas: *vata*, *pitta*, and *kapha*. The conversation between the doshas in our bodies, our daily activities, and the natural world around us inform and guide our wellness. These will be described in detail in chapters 6 and 7, with more tools listed in the Resources for Further Study section at the back of the book.

The Path of Balance

Even though it was written for monastics, the Rule has been a social and spiritual influence for more than 1,500 years. Attention to God's presence in all things, the importance of right relationship, stability, listening, growth, hospitality, rhythms, silence, and sabbath: these themes transcend the walls of the monastery. Anyone can apply these underlying concepts to daily life. The temptation to say that it is easier to live them out within the confines of a cloister is to dismiss the shared challenges of being human. Yes, it may be less difficult for a monk or nun to pause and pray the psalms and liturgies seven times a day than it is for a layperson, but is it any easier to focus on the Divine in the moment?

Balanced living in spirit, mind, and body is a dynamic conversation between steadiness and motion, work and prayer, sound and silence, activity and rest. Study and application of the balancing way of Benedictine spirituality and yoga are useful markers on the path. Their wisdom has endured the test of time with its evolving cultural norms, politics, theology, technology, and medicine precisely because these traditions bring a steadying dialogue within an ever-changing world.

If you are new to Benedictine spirituality, yoga, or Ayurveda, or if any of the ideas and practices in this book feel foreign, I encourage you to approach them with an open mind and the Benedictine principles of listening and growth. We don't know what we don't know. The path of balance invites us to be curious, exploratory, and receptive to God's call in the here and now.

In the prologue to the Rule, Benedict quotes Jesus's words: "Run while you have the light of life, that the darkness of death may not overtake you" (John 12:35). The first Yoga Sutra reads, "Now is the exposition of yoga." The time is now. Balance is not an elusive goal. The path of balance is like God: ever present and in all places. All we must do is shift our attention to see it and welcome it more fully into our hearts and lives. In this moment. Now.

Humility
The Fertile Ground

Sisters and brothers, divine Scripture calls to us saying,

"Whoever exalt themselves shall be humbled,

and whoever humble themselves shall be exalted."

—St. Benedict and Luke 14:11

For days I was irritated that a colleague had not given me some notes I'd requested weeks earlier. When I saw him as we were both leaving for the day, I casually and cheerfully said, "Hey, can you give me those notes?"

"I already did. I put them in your box right after you emailed me."

"Oh. They're not there. I'll have to look around."

The next morning as I was getting my son ready for school and myself ready for work, I suddenly remembered taking the papers from my box, reading and making notes, punching holes, and filing them in the binder. In that remembering, I recognized just how overworked and overcommitted I had become. Despite my claims to the contrary, I did not have everything under control. I could not do all that was being asked of me. In the hubris of my independence, I had lost touch with the fertile ground of balance.

That fertile ground is the Benedictine way of humility.

Humility is the practice of being in right relationship with God, ourselves, and one another. It is a quietness of heart and freedom of breath that exists when we remember we are not in charge of everyone and everything around us. It is a wellspring of moderation that balances our need to work, rest, play, pray, engage, and release.

In yoga this moderation is called *brahmacharya*. Brahmacharya means "walk with God." It also means continence, or moderation. Patanjali's Yoga Sutra says, "When the practitioner is firmly established in continence, knowledge, and vigor, valor and energy flow to her." When we practice moderation, a vitality of mind, body, and spirit returns to the places that were once depleted by too much—or perhaps too little—effort. When we practice moderation, we are walking with a power greater than ourselves, because we are no longer trying to consume or control out of fear. Without humility and moderation, we cannot possibly hope to change our unintentional, unbalanced, self-destructive ways of being.

Benedict's treatise on humility was a radical alternative to the world of excess, toxic power, privilege, and exploitation that characterized the declining Roman Empire in which he lived. The intent of practicing humility was to strip oneself of false pretense and become more Christlike: to create space within one's self to be a welcoming, loving presence for others and to be a servant of God.

Unfortunately, the original beauty of humility was warped into a tool for oppression. Humility often equated to the subservience of women to men and enslaved people to masters. Self-flagellation—whether chosen or directed by those in authority—became at times an outward humiliation intended to demonstrate humility before God without necessarily bringing about a change of heart. As such, our first reaction to the notion of humility is often one of aversion.

On this path of balance, we are invited to reclaim the practice of humility as one in which we can gently and lovingly be reminded that we are not alone. We are not alone in our arrogance, our overwork, our fatigue. We are not alone in our gifts, our joys, our goodness. We are an essential thread in the tapestry of life, woven together with all the other messy threads in the beauty of creation.

Placing ourselves on the path of humility means both grounding and surrender. Humility is derived from the Latin *humus*, which means "earth." Through humility, we root ourselves in God, who nourishes, sustains, and gives us life. Through humility we are able to see and surrender our ways of being that lead to imbalance.

The Twelve Stages of Humility

In the Rule, Benedict outlines twelve stages of humility, or twelve ways of approaching life with a spirit of moderation and right relationship. In the Yoga Sutras, there are five moral precepts—*yamas*—and five ethical precepts—*niyamas*—that lay the foundation for a yogic life. In *Meditations from the Mat*, yoga teachers Rolf Gates and Katrina Kenison describe them as the bedrock of "spirituality in action" and "sustainers of a life based on love." These principles compose the foundation of the rest of the practice, or *abhyasa*. Gates and Kenison go on to write, "Abhyasa refers not only to yogic practice but also to the attitude with which a practice is approached. Abhyasa is unconditional. It is the dedicated, unswerving application of what you believe in."

I see Benedict's stages of humility in conversation with the yamas and niyamas. They reinforce his vision of humility in action. The yamas and niyamas are often presented in a linear manner, as outlined in the preceding chapter and in the Yoga Sutra. The connections I make in the following paragraphs do not follow this linear approach but rather draw on their essential principles as they relate to humility.

The first stage of humility is to keep the focus of life on the sacred by maintaining a reverence for the world God created and by loving the God of Creation. Moving our focus beyond ourselves as the center of the universe is a challenge. The yama of *ahimsa*—or that which is non-harming or life-affirming—brings us back to an affirmation of the God-given world.

The second stage of humility is to surrender our will and let go of our need to have things our own way. *Ishvara pranidhana*—surrender to God—leads us to the place where our deepest desires bring great good in the world. These are not desires for more and better, for success and esteem, or for the transient wants of the day. The seeming contradiction here is that by surrendering our timelines and plans, we create room for God's desire that we live in the fullness of who we were created to be.

The third and fourth stages of humility are about knowing ourselves well. Similarly, the niyama of *svadhyaya* is the call to study the world, the Divine, and our relationship to it with depth and authenticity. Here we become honest about our limitations, frailties, insecurities, strengths. We learn to have patience with ourselves and our circumstances, choosing not to aggrandize or succumb to a seductive sense of guilt. Knowing ourselves well, we are able to practice perseverance in the face of difficulty because we know that we are not in this alone. We are not the only ones who struggle, and we can rely on our community and God to pick us up when we are stuck in cycles of despair.

The fifth stage of humility is rigorous honesty about our actions and motivations. We practice the yama of *satya*, or truth. This is where we have the opportunity to let go of the facades we build to protect ourselves from criticism and the persistent fear and anxiety that we are not good enough. With satya and the fifth stage of humility, we recognize the truth of our humanity in all its foibles and graces.

The sixth stage of humility is to practice contentment, or *santosha*. Life often doesn't go the way we plan or desire. Trials happen—some great, some small. It is our response to our circumstances that makes all the difference.

The seventh stage is knowing our own proportionality. We are neither good nor bad—neither the center of the universe nor its most outlying periphery. We are part of the matrix of life, with God as the center. This stage is another reiteration of satya and svadhyaya: truth and study of Self and the sacred.

The eighth and ninth stages of humility bring us deeper into relationship with community through obedience and guidance from others and the practice of nonjudgment. This is the beginning of *aparigraha*: non-clinging or letting go. Letting go of our assumptions that we know what is best for ourselves and the people around us. Letting go of the need to place others in rigid boxes that define who they are before we even get a chance to know them. Further, we are called to practice nonjudgment of ourselves, so that once again we see who God lovingly created us to be.

The tenth and eleventh stages of humility bring us into empathy and moderation of speech, as we discern what is humorous and what is cruel. We become able to listen and respond rather than blather on about our own worlds. We are invited to return to the practice of ahimsa, by not harming others with our attitudes and actions, and to the practice of brahmacharya, or remaining moderate in how we speak and act.

The twelfth stage of humility is to practice all of these principles with devotion so they become our first instinct. This requires *tapas*, or burning zeal in practice. We so long to live and walk in love that we do what we can, with the support of those around us and with reliance on Grace to keep us going. In this way, humility can become the very fabric of our days.

These are not easy tasks. We cannot do them alone, because they all exist in relationship. Our communities give us the landscape in which to navigate this spiritual orientation and growth. Those to whom we belong—in families and friendships, churches and other communities of faith and practice—afford us the honor of pursuing humility together.

Approaching change—whether change of heart, mind, routine, diet, work, or relationship—with humility helps us remember that we are held and encouraged by a Divine Power greater than ourselves. We are loved into positive ways of being. Humility invites us to let go of our perfectionism and need to control, and open to the joy of beginning and failing and beginning again.

As we humbly seek to make changes that reorient us toward balance, two key slogans borrowed from the twelve-step recovery programs are of use: "Easy does it," and "Progress, not perfection."

Easy Does It

When I get to work on Monday morning, the first thing I do is take out my planner and make notes for the week ahead. I list all the tasks and projects that I need to get done—and because color makes me happy, I use highlighters to color-code my time blocks. Some weeks, especially those with appointments that take me away from work, feel like too much, and I am overwhelmed before the week begins. There's a small box at the top of my weekly page labeled "Focus for this week." My first thought of what to write there is always "Just get through." But my second thought is often "Easy does it."

I know from experience in work and in my yoga practice that when I approach my schedule, a project, or an asana with gentleness, I am more productive, feel more nourished, and generally enjoy life more than when I push or rush. Practicing "Easy does it" is a way for me to get out of my arrogant need to be perfect and in control and step into the care of a loving God. Practicing "Easy does it" is a small, simple way of living the Benedictine way of humility.

Here is an example of this perspective in a yoga practice. I wake up and unroll my yoga mat. I sit, breathe, and check in with my energy. How much do I have? What is the quality? Do I feel groggy, lethargic, excited, joyful? More often than not, I come to a practice from a place of unease and agitation. I start slow: Child's Pose with a twist, Cat-Cow tilts on hands and knees, a long and luxurious Downward-Facing Dog. Then I move into basic Sun Salutations with lunge variations. If my energy is clearing and growing, I might pick up the pace, perhaps moving into more challenging or advanced postures. If I'm still feeling low, I may slow down, do a smaller version of an asana shape, or take the entire practice to the floor for seated forward folds and twists.

Whatever the speed, intensity, or degree of difficulty in my practice, my aim is always to approach it with ease. Easy does it. This is where breathing comes in. Allowing movement to follow in the wake of the breath is the basic unit of each posture. It is humility embodied, because each action is a response to a deeper wisdom.

Off the mat, "Easy does it" may look like shifting (or canceling) appointments to free up time, taking a walk outside at lunch, or cooking a simple dinner. It may mean texting with a friend to tell her I am frightened and receive a comforting and simple reminder to breathe, or it may mean consciously slowing my steps as I walk.

All these measures help return me to balance because they are small, easy-to-implement actions that diffuse overstimulation. There's nothing grandiose about rescheduling a doctor's appointment, having healthy breakfast food with fruit for dinner, or texting a friend. Yet such minute shifts reflect an inner posture of humility that opens a path for God to enter and direct my life.

When we're making changes in response to feelings of imbalance and unease, it is helpful to go slow. Small actions over a sustained period of time have more staying power than grand gestures that crash and lead to disheartening returns to our destructive habits.

As you move through the chapters and wellness exercises in this book, I invite you to take it easy. Choose one or two practices that seem the most manageable and start there before attempting to implement others. Proceed with the knowledge that you will fail often and that you will find yourself right back in patterns of overwhelm and fatigue. Benedict knew this, and he advised his monks gently and lovingly to begin again. (This is a process called *conversatio morum*, which we will look at in chapter 4.) It's okay to fail. Balance is a dynamic conversation. It requires the humility to see and accept our habitual modes of imbalance and respond with small, manageable action. It requires the second slogan borrowed from twelve-step programs: "Progress, not perfection."

Progress, Not Perfection

Benedict knew that as humans we are fallible, fickle beings, prone to lofty ideals and not so great at follow-through. He knew this and made room for it in the

Rule. Benedict encouraged his monks to recognize their failures and each time return with humility to God, who has the power to bring about the change of heart and action we seek.

In the fall of my senior year in college, I had an art history paper due and was overwhelmed by my waitressing job and coursework. I found myself anxious and stressed about how I was going to get the paper done on time given my other commitments. One rainy day when I was driving around town, however, it occurred to me that I had never once turned an assignment in late. There was no need to worry about my schedule. I would complete the assignment on time.

That moment was so profound, so visceral, that whenever I feel nervous about a deadline now, I breathe and picture myself in my car on that day. I see the gray sky, hear the rain on the windshield, and listen to the soft whisper reminding me that all will get done because I know how to back off. I know how to create space. I know how to let God lead the way.

If I stick to the perception that after that moment in college I will never again feel overwhelmed by a deadline, I set myself up for disappointment. I am often overwhelmed. I nearly always stress about deadlines. Yet the progress is that I can now recognize that I'm in a space of imbalance and return to the lesson learned in college. Now I can shift from saying "I've *got* to get this done" to "God, guide my schedule and my work." The progress is that I can laugh instead of berate myself for being in a state of anxiety. Again.

"Progress, not perfection" is an essential ally on the path of balance, because it frees us of the hubris that we can be flawless or do everything all on our own. Humility recognizes that the only perfection we can achieve is to be authentically who we are, imperfections and all, while continuing to embrace the evolving process of trying, failing, and beginning again. We can only do this with the help of a Higher Power.

Questions for Reflection

- What is your first response to "humility"? Has the idea of humility been used to demean you? If so, how might you reframe it in the Benedictine way of quietness of heart and relationship with God?

- Which of the twelve stages of humility, and its corresponding yama and niyama, calls out to you the most?

- How does your body feel when you consider "Easy does it" and "Progress, not perfection"? What happens to your breath? Does it constrict, slow, release, open?

- Looking at your commitments for the week, where and how can you make space for God to guide you?

- How does it feel to know you will probably slide right back into your old patterns but always have the opportunity to try again, knowing you are gently loved along the way?

Wellness Practice: Take a Contemplative Walk

It is easy to overcomplicate things. We read and write treatises on how to move the body for optimal efficiency, weight loss, and form. Power walk for three minutes, slow down for one, pause for thirty seconds, repeat. Throw in some jumping jacks or a short sprint to optimize cardiovascular health. As a longtime yogi, I know there is benefit to the study and analysis of movement. Yet sometimes it is important just to move without overanalyzing.

A contemplative walk is an invitation to retreat from the need to control or force a solution and settle into the quiet partnership found in Benedictine humility. Whenever possible, I take a walk outside after lunch. Whether my pace is fast or slow, I use this time to breathe and observe the world around me: light filtered through the trees, crows and hawks flying over the creek, roots pushing up through the pavement. Gentle attention to the comings and goings of nature, to the sound of my feet and my breath, moves me out of an overactive mode of trying to perfectly sort a million pieces of data from my day and puts me again in right relationship with God, myself, and the world. Solutions to problems appear. My head is not quite as a hot. Dizziness from staring at the computer abates. I feel rebalanced.

The key to a contemplative walk is not so much in the pacing, though I personally find it helps to slow down, but rather in attention. It takes time to to calm the nerves. In paying attention to the flow of your thoughts, the feeling of the air against your skin, the animals that show up, the people who pass by, the body and mind move from a state of overstimulation into a more comfortable rhythm.

Make time this week—ten minutes, twenty minutes, or whatever amount of time you can find—to take a contemplative walk outside. You can do this solo or with a friend. Let go of any need for it to be a body-shaping, calorie-burning exercise for the day. As you put one foot in front of the other, notice the world around you. What colors do you see? Are there trees, flowers, desert? How does the air feel? What sound do your feet make as you walk? What animals do you see? You don't have to name everything you see, although you can; simply let yourself observe. Remember that you too are a part of the creation you see all around you.

Meditation: The Fertile Ground

Sit in a comfortable seat with your spine erect. Welcome and observe a few rounds of natural breath. As you draw your attention inward, start to picture yourself in your favorite outdoor space: a garden, a forest, by the water, in the desert, on a mountain. Make it vivid. What vegetation surrounds you? What animals are with you? Feel a sweet, warm air around you, perhaps a gentle breeze brushing against your skin. Let your inner senses be flooded with the beauty of the world around you.

Walk around this space, and then find a comfortable place to sit or lie down on the earth. Feel yourself supported by the earth beneath you. Watch how the world around you moves about its business without any direction or effort on your part. The animals find their food. The birds sing and the clouds float across the sky. Notice that you too are a part of this creation. You breathe in the air, and as you exhale, your breath feeds the green things around you.

Begin to imagine roots growing from your spine, down though your tailbone and into the earth. Feel nourishment rising up from the earth to meet you as you release down into its support. You are part of the sacred world—instrumental but not in charge.

Rest in this space for some time. When you are ready, welcome in a few deep breaths and then open your eyes.

Asana Practice: Moving with the Breath

We begin our movement practice with postures that awaken the spine and focus on aligning movement with breath. The first action of any pose is to breathe. When we consciously invite the breath to come before the movement, we open to the guidance of Spirit. Letting the breath lead the way is an embodied demonstration of humility. We step away from the need to push our way through life, to shapeshift mindlessly from one pose to the next, and we place ourselves more fully in the currents of Grace.

The asanas in this sequence on humility form the building blocks for the asanas and sequences throughout the rest of the book. I encourage you to take your time. Savor these gentle movements, and focus on allowing your breath to let you know when it is time to move to the next pose and when it is time to stay still. Easy does it.

Apanasana: Knees-to-Chest Pose

Lie down on your back with your knees bent and your feet on the floor. Bring your hands to your abdomen and breathe. Feel the rise and fall of your belly as you inhale and exhale. Welcome a soft ease as you settle into the support of the ground beneath you. Keep your spine neutral so there is a gentle, natural curve in your lower back.

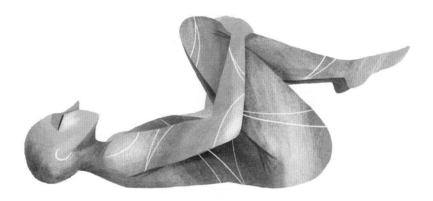

After a few rounds of breath, draw your knees in toward your chest and hug your shins with your hands. You may stay still here as you breathe or begin to rock from side to side. Go slow. There is no need to rush. The currents of Grace flow sweetly and in their own time.

If you'd like, you may create small, circular movements with your legs that initiate from the tops of your thighs. This action releases gripping in the hips and opens the pathways for the grounding, downward flow of *prana*, or life energy.

Continue to breathe and move in a way that feels easeful. When you are ready, let go of your shins and lower your feet to the floor.

Sucirandhrasana: Eye of the Needle Pose

Lying on your back with your pelvis neutral, breathe, lift your right foot, and cross your ankle over your left thigh. You may stay just like this or place your right hand gently on your right thigh to create a mental connection from the periphery of your body to the core. Breathe and feel the soft sensation in your outer hips and belly. This may be plenty.

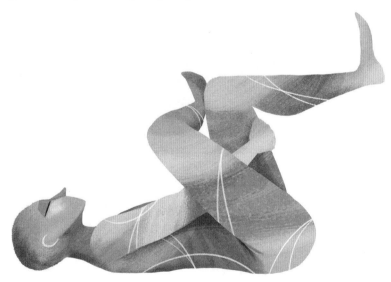

If you feel you have the mobility to move further, lift your left foot off the floor and draw your knees in toward your chest. Thread your right hand between your legs and hold the back of your left thigh. Relax your shoulders and keep your head resting on the floor.

Allow your breath to be your guide. If bringing your knees close to your chest causes constriction in your breathing, tightness in your tummy, or tension in your neck, back off, perhaps placing your left foot back on the floor. There is no prize for creating this shape. The only goal of this asana, and of any asana, is to align your body with your breath and, in doing so, to align your actions with the prompting of the Divine.

After five to seven rounds of breath, or however many feel comfortable, place your feet back on the floor. Repeat this posture on the second side by crossing your left ankle over your right thigh.

When you are done, draw both knees in toward your chest and roll to one side. Pause there for a full breath cycle and then press up to a comfortable sitting position.

Marjaryasana–Bitilasana: Cat Pose–Cow Pose

Come to what we call a table-top position: kneel on all fours with your knees under your hips and hands under your shoulders. Widen your feet to be hip-width distance apart, and rotate your wrists so their creases are parallel to the front of your mat. Allow your fingers to gently spread. This will help soften your shoulders.

If you have knee pain, place a blanket or small towel under your knees. If you have wrist pain, place a small, rolled towel under the base of your palm to reduce the angle of bend in your wrists.

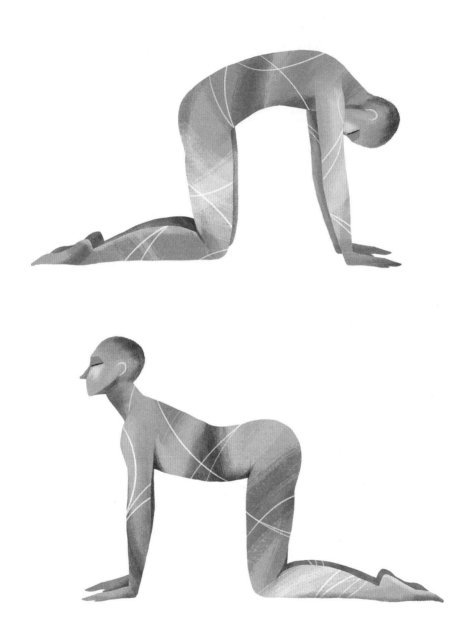

Return to an awareness of your breath. As you inhale, begin to tip your tailbone toward the backs of your knees and round your back upward. Let your head release downward. This is Cat Pose. As you exhale, tip your pelvis forward to melt your belly and chest toward the floor. Lift your head as your chest expands. This is Cow Pose.

Continue to flow between arching and releasing your back. Let each movement follow in the wake of your breath. Initiate the action from the tilt in your pelvis rather than the middle of your back. This is growing the pose from the ground up. Only round to the point of gentle sensation. While it may feel good to push into an extreme arch in either pose, it is better to stay small and engaged rather than big and forced. Moving within a smaller range of motion is an excellent way to practice right relationship and humility.

Move through this flow, back and forth between Cat and Cow, for several rounds of breath. Then return to a neutral spine.

Balasana: Child's Pose

Starting from table-top position on your hands and knees, bring your feet together and widen your knees a few inches apart. Breathe and stretch back so your hips sit on or near your heels. You may keep your arms extended or place them alongside your hips.

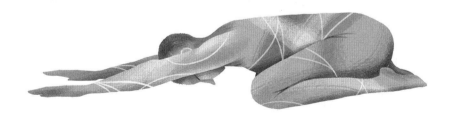

This posture is also considered a deep *pranam*, or position of prayer and greeting.

As you inhale, welcome in the wellspring of the Divine that nurtures and sustains you. As you exhale, offer a prayer to let go of your need to control. Connect this intention of humility before God to the rhythms of the body, and with each inhale, feel the gentle expansion in the back of your ribs and the sensation and space between your vertebrae. With each exhale, let your belly relax. Many of us hold unconscious tension in the abdomen as a result of trying too hard to look a certain way. Give yourself permission to relax into your body as it is. I know this may be difficult. Let your breath be your guide.

Adho Mukha Svanasana: Downward-Facing Dog Pose

If your arms were by your sides in Child's Pose, extend them over your head now. Place your palms on the mat shoulder-width distance apart or slightly wider.

Downward-Facing Dog is a pose that builds strength, and it may take some time to be able to hold it for more than a breath or two. Go easy on yourself. If you have wrist or shoulder injuries, check with your health-care provider before you proceed. You may also place a small folded dish towel or washcloth under the base of your palms to elevate and reduce the angle of bend in your wrists. Child's Pose with arms extended is also a beautiful option if Downward-Facing Dog is too rigorous. You can also do Downward-Facing Dog with your hands on the seat or back of a chair, or shoulder height at the wall.

From Child's Pose, tuck your toes and bring your knees hip-width distance apart.

Breathe. Check to see that your hands are shoulder-width distance apart, wrist creases parallel to the front of the mat and fingers gently spread.

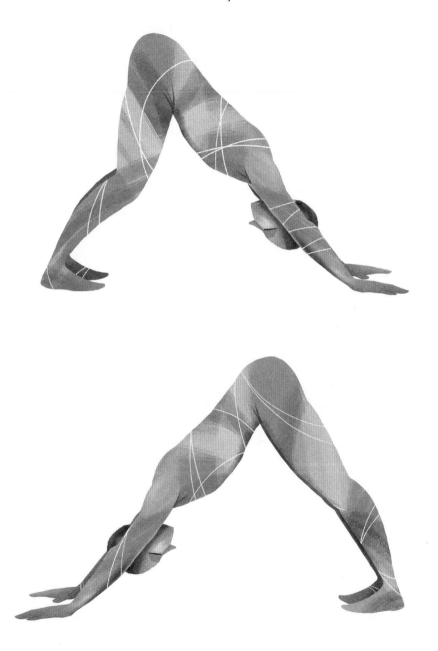

Inhale and press the inner and outer edges of your hands and finger pads into the mat to evenly engage the muscles of your arms, and root into the support of the ground. Exhale.

On your next inhale, lift your knees off the floor and reach your hips to the sky. Keeping your knees bent, exhale and soften the space between the back of your shoulder blades.

Stay in this pose, the bent-knee Downward-Facing Dog, for a breath or two. As you breathe, firm your arms toward the midline as though there were magnets along the inseam of your arms.

Begin to push your thighs back and straighten your legs. This is Downward-Facing Dog. But here is another opportunity to embody humility: bring your attention to your lower back. If you feel your lower back round as it did in the Cat Pose, bend your knees again. This will release overeffort in the hamstrings and help maintain a healthy, neutral curve in your lower back.

As you inhale, draw energy from the ground under your hands and feet up your arms and legs and into the space between your shoulder blades. This is the center of gravity in your pose, also known as the back of your energetic heart. Welcoming in the power of the breath here demonstrates a willingness to humbly engage with the Divine. With your exhale, release your effort out from your heart through your spine, arms, and legs. Let your heels release toward the floor. They don't need to touch the floor; simply allow gravity to support a downward flow and release. With each drawing in, you open to a power greater than yourself. With each extension back out, you humbly follow the guidance of a Higher Power.

Stay in Downward-Facing Dog for three to seven breaths. But again, if you can only do one breath, wonderful. If you are unable to support yourself in Downward-Facing Dog, continue with Child's Pose or a modification at the wall.

You can still explore the dynamic of drawing in and extending out of humble opening and right action.

Uttanasana: Standing Forward Fold Pose

Now, from Downward-Facing Dog or a modification of this pose, inhale, walk your feet toward your hands, and come into a Standing Forward Fold. Give a slight bend to your knees to prevent hyperextension and to offer a little more ease to tight hamstrings.

Bring your hands to your legs, a block in front of your feet, or the floor. Whatever you can comfortably reach will work. You may even wrap your hands around the backs of your legs or hold your forearms in front of your shins. However you choose to place your hands, be sure they make contact with something tangible, be it another part of your body, a prop, or the floor. This will help maintain a subtle yet powerful connection to the core and enhance the feeling of grounding and release.

Breathe in and gently lift your toes to engage the muscles evenly on all four sides of your legs. Breathe out and extend from your pelvis down to the ground, rooting into the support of the Divine.

Stay here for three to five breaths, or however long you feel comfortable.

Tadasana: Mountain Pose

From Standing Forward Fold, inhale; press your feet into the floor and bring your hands to your hips. Exhale. Staying strong and rooted through your legs, inhale and lift your torso to rise up to standing. As you breathe, release your arms down by your sides.

Stand tall and breathe. Maintain gentle engagement in your legs and torso while releasing any overeffort or bracing in your gluteal muscles and belly. With each inhale, become aware of a light lift in your chest as you invite Divine guidance into your life. With each exhale, soften your shoulders and settle into that higher wisdom.

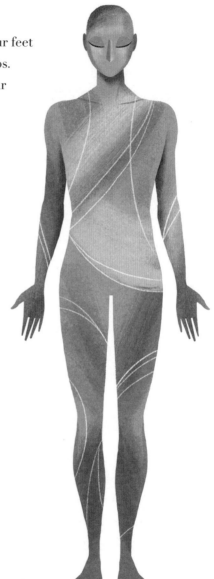

CHAPTER

3

Obedience
Listening to the Guide

Listen carefully, my child, to my instructions and attend to them with the ear of your heart. This is advice from one who loves you; welcome it and faithfully put it into practice.

—St. Benedict

I am often amazed when my young child listens to—and obeys—my instructions. Many times it is a struggle to get him to pay attention and respond as directed, but frequently he does hear and follow through. A "no" from me is his least favorite answer to a request, but eventually, sometimes after a bit of a tantrum, he accepts my authority as his mother and moves on. I hope that he is obedient because he knows I love him unconditionally and would never do anything to intentionally break his free, wild, and wonderful spirit. I hope that he knows I simply want to help him grow into a kind, loving, and capable adult, secure in the knowledge that his gifts have a place in this world.

And so it is with God.

The very first word of Benedict's Rule is "listen." Listen to these words with your whole being, Benedict tells us; "attend to them with the ear of your heart." Know they come from a place of love.

Listening is an action-oriented skill. We open ourselves enough to hear what is being said or asked and then choose how to respond. In *Seeking God: The Way of St. Benedict*, Esther de Waal writes that the response is critical, because it takes listening beyond the intellect and into lived action.

Yoga asanas are a particularly powerful training ground for mindful, active listening. Time on the mat is dedicated to call and response. Bodily sensation arises as we move and breathe and choose how to interact with or ignore signals of tension, weakness, or pain in our efforts to find balanced action. A constriction in the belly may be a prompt to relax the diaphragm. A hardening in the hips could indicate the need to back out of the shape just enough to engage the core. Pose after pose, we meet the language of the body and are invited to listen and grow, or ignore and stagnate.

This same call-and-response pattern within our bodies happens off the mat as well. Maybe you are sitting at your desk when you notice a pain in your neck, so you roll your head from side to side. Perhaps you feel a strain in your back, and adjust your seat or pause and take a break from the task at hand. Practicing obedience is responding to the call of the moment with attention and intention.

Deep, active listening is central to both yoga and the Benedictine Way. Listening calls us out of habitual self-centeredness and destructive patterns and into healthy relationship with our bodies, ourselves, and our community.

Obedience is one of the vows taken by Benedictine monks when they enter the monastery. "Obedience is derived from the Latin *oboedire*, which shares its root with *audire*, which means 'to hear,'" writes de Waal. Benedict places significant emphasis on surrendering self-will in favor of obedience to God. Yet Benedictine obedience is not about a simplistic or mechanical yes to instruction. Nor is it about abandoning oneself and one's God-given gifts in the world in favor of false austerity. De Waal goes on to write that Benedict asks his monks to give up *possessive* will, not *free* will, which is the greatest of gifts. Our free will gives us a choice in each moment: to either be in open, loving relationship with Grace or else to be mired in a tiresome, destructive, and shallow experience of life.

"The labor of obedience will bring you back to God," Benedict writes in the prologue. The yogic complement to Benedictine obedience is *ishvara pranidhana:* surrender to God. Surrendering to God may feel like a monumental undertaking. Letting go of our own agenda runs counter to our habits of self-reliance and goal-setting. Like the yoga sages, Benedict is aware of how difficult the path is. Surrendering self-centered desire in favor of obedience to a higher wisdom demands much stripping of who we think we are and what we should be doing in the world. On the other hand, just as a child can trust a loving parent's instructions, you can be assured that surrender and obedience to Divine Will is a resounding yes to becoming the person who a loving God created you to be.

Like every other part of the path of balance, obedient surrender is lived one small step at a time. Each moment offers the invitation to listen to the call of God and respond from a place of integrity.

For instance, perhaps you planned to take a walk or get on the yoga mat or meditate or pray, but when the time comes, you just don't feel like it. You know your body and spirit are crying out for this kind of practice, but your mind would rather be engaged in ticking off items on your to-do list. Despite this struggle, you go on your walk, step on the mat, or sit for meditation or prayer anyway. In doing so, you have listened to the call of a greater wisdom, surrendered your task-focused agenda, and followed the will of the Spirit. Your efforts are rewarded with more clarity of thought, vibrancy in your body, and perhaps a deep sense of connection and equanimity. This is listening and obedience in action.

Listening for the Season

Finding balance means we must first locate those parts of ourselves that feel unbalanced. Through deep listening we can name the ways of living that run counter to God's call for us. Through deep listening we acknowledge the patterns and behaviors in our lives that do not provide nourishment, and we can claim the wisdom of the heart, mind, and body that points us toward balance and well-being.

I'm a dreamer. There is so much I want to do and study in my lifetime. The temptation is to want to do all of it now, out of fear that otherwise I never will. Benedict tasks us to "Keep death daily before your eyes," and "Run while you have the light of life." This is not, however, a call to reactive, frantic, overscheduled living. It is a call to deeply listen to the Spirit's prompting via a thoughtful, lived response.

The first sutra in the *Yoga Sutras of Patanjali* reads: "Now is the exposition, practice, and study of yoga." The time is now. Don't delay your commitment to spiritual study and action, but recognize that it is a practice, something to be done over and over again throughout the seasons of life.

One of the questions that orients me toward balanced living is "What season of life am I in, and what does that mean for now, for today?" As we do when we observe the rhythms of the earth, we can begin to learn from the wisdom of now. The sun rises and the sun sets. The summer is plentiful with fruit and heat. The winter is cold and dormant. Not everything happens at once, and yet each now is a complete expression of its own moment in time.

When we're feeling out of balance, often it is because we are not responding to the season of now. We're trying to cram too much into a day, a week, a year. We're not listening to the needs of the body and the wisdom of the heart. Obedience to the call for balanced living requires an honest reckoning with the current season of life. Having unrealistic expectations of what we can do in this space and time sets us up for fatigue and a nagging sense that we aren't good enough at this life and spirituality business.

A busy parent of young children, for example, may be thwarted by a child's uncanny ability to need something at the very moment the parent sits down to meditate. For such a parent, it may not be the season for prolonged daily meditation. Perhaps this season is an invitation to practice deep listening and loving response to the child at hand while finding other ways to carve out time for more realistic self-care.

A retiree may find that, after decades of work, settling in to a new and fulfilling rhythm requires a shift in the definition of a productive and meaningful day. Perhaps, after years of a schedule ruled by the demands of others, this season of life affords time and space to listen.

Seasonal living is ripe with gifts of the Spirit. Take time to listen to the call of life as it is today. Responding accordingly is a positive and powerful step on the path of sacred balance.

Obedience in Community

A key component of deep listening and obedience is gathering wisdom from a support system. God speaks to us in many ways, and Benedict is adamant that obedience happens in community. The oblate may not understand why the abbot or abbess is instructing a particular action. But having taken a vow of obedience, she carries it out anyway, trusting that guidance is in her best interest.

This is why we have teachers, mentors, trusted friends, and loved ones. In yoga, it is vital to have instruction from someone who has studied and is a little further ahead on the path. This keeps us safe as we begin or experiment with new ways of approaching familiar poses and breath practices. It is also important to have a community of practitioners—even if it's just a community of one or two other people—with whom to connect and share experience, and to support along the way.

We don't know what we don't know. Our kindred on the path to sacred balance help us listen to our lives and discern what God calls us to do. They help us navigate the season of now and hold loving space for us to choose our response.

At the same time, obedience calls us beyond being a mere recipient of the wisdom and guidance of others. We are also charged with the important work of shepherding others along their paths. Inviting the obedience of those whose spheres we inhabit isn't about advice-giving or control. It is about opening ourselves to become a loving presence and safe harbor for the members of our community to explore the call in their own lives. We listen and respond with love. Through obedience to others and their obedience to us, we rise to the commitments we make to friends and relatives, church family, chosen family, yoga community, and work colleagues.

Going further, we are also called to obedient listening and response to communities beyond our own. We are called to care for the sick, the stranger, the refugee, the immigrant, the acquaintance who just lost her job. How we go about living God's call to be in ever-widening circles of community looks different for each of us, depending on our gifts and our season of life.

In the Jewish tradition there is a practice of taking care of one's immediate family before the extended family, and then broadening out to one's religious community, local town, state, country, and global society. Communities beyond our own are to be seen, listened to, and responded to as an extension of getting our own house in order.

My father, who is an Episcopal priest, has always been clear when teaching on the practice of tithing: if you can't afford to buy your child food or shoes, perhaps you are not called to tithe money in this season of life. Rather, the call to be obedient may be to give your time or talents to the community while stewarding your treasure for the immediate needs of your family. Balanced obedience looks different for each of us at every stage and season of our lives.

For those who, like me, are more introverted and tend to keep our own counsel, some levels of obedience can be a challenge. I am good at holding space for others to explore their own lives but not so great at letting others help me explore mine. It has taken years for me to cultivate close friendships with people I trust and with whom I can share my innermost self. A few years ago I was discerning a rather substantial redirection in my life when I took a leap of faith and reached out to a priest, who agreed to act as my spiritual director for a year. She listened, offered context in which to navigate my inquiry, gave honest and direct feedback, and was there for me when I decided how to act upon the ways we heard God moving in my life. I could not have explored that moment without her and a handful of others in my community. Obeying God's call for my life during that season was one of the most difficult, frightening, and ultimately liberating things I have ever done. It has led to grace beyond measure. Of my own accord, I might not have responded as I did but might instead have remained in a situation that grew increasingly toxic. With the help and support of community, I was able to choose otherwise.

That is the power of obedience in community. It is in the context of relationship that we grow and help others do the same.

Questions for Reflection

- What season of life are you in? What adjectives would you use to describe it?

- What activities or dreams are you trying to squeeze into this season of life that may be better suited for another?

- What activities or dreams may it be time to say yes to?

- What communities do you inhabit?

- How do you practice obedience within the framework of community? Whom do you reach out to for support? For whom do you stand as a compassionate presence?

- How else do you practice obedience?

Wellness Practice: Practice Sacred Reading

Lectio divina means "sacred reading," and as a practice, it can prompt deep listening and an authentic response to the invitation of Spirit, bringing comfort when needed and challenge when vital. Lectio is the practice of engaging with a short text through four specific movements that bring us out of a mere analytical relationship with words and into a heart language of call and response. The four primary movements of lectio are read, reflect, respond, and rest. Benedict required the monks to spend large portions of the day praying lectio with Scripture as a way to "listen with the ears of the heart." Scripture was not to be learned by rote and regurgitated at opportune moments. Scripture was to be an encounter that led to transformation and a deeper life in Christ.

Though a practice rooted in biblical study, lectio can be done with any text that moves you—a poem, a song, a line from a film, even an image. For years I practiced lectio with a secular daily reader that I turn to often. Even now I find each encounter with that text provides fresh challenge and new wisdom. I am not the same person I was the first time I read a particular passage. It had time to work in me, and now I can listen anew.

In an ideal world, we would set aside ten to fifteen minutes or more each day for lectio. It takes time to grow quiet enough to listen beyond intellect. We may want to incorporate lectio but those moments are just too difficult to find. If that is the case, we can explore creative ways to adapt the practice, such as inviting an image or word to shimmer in our awareness while on a contemplative walk. Or we could write down a text on an index card, or in a note on a cell phone, and return to it several times throughout the day. Lectio can also be done in a partnership or group setting, such as a Bible or book study. For me, group study has been the most enriching experience of lectio, because I am able to move beyond my own assumptions and bias and open myself to a different perspective.

I invite you to use the text below as a starting point for your lectio practice, or you could choose one of your own. It is important to keep the text relatively short, so your attention can home in on the wisdom being offered in the moment.

> "You have made the moon to mark the seasons; the sun knows
> its time for setting." (Psalm 104:19 NRSV)

Lectio: Reading and Listening

Welcome a few breaths to center yourself and create an inner environment of receptivity. Read through the text one time, out loud if possible. As your eyes move over the words, watch for a word or phrase that shimmers. Allow yourself to be drawn to a small portion of the passage. Pause. Read the text a second time. What stands out to you now? Is it the same word or phrase from the initial reading, or is it something new? As Cynthia Bourgeault writes in *The Wisdom Jesus*, "The important point is not *what* you're struck by, but *that* you're struck by it—that is, your willingness to trust that as you open to the passage in this deeply listening and receptive way, something will indeed be calling. Stick with it; follow its lead." Without overanalysis, stay with this word or phrase as you move onto the next stage of lectio.

Meditatio: Reflecting

Remain quiet and let the word or phrase that shimmered stay in your awareness. Allow it to unfold in your imagination, stimulating thoughts and associations from your life. What images or memories arise? How might this small segment of the reading relate to your life today?

Oratio: Prayer and Response

As you reflect on the word or passage that shimmered for you, listen for its invitation. Feel your feelings as you encounter the text. Notice if the word brings you comfort. If so, how? Does the passage trigger or challenge you in some way? If so, what is being triggered? If you like to journal, take this as a good opportunity to free-write about the passage.

Contemplatio: Resting in God

Let go of the word or phrase and let yourself breathe. Open to a quiet space where you are neither speaking nor actively listening, but just resting. Like letting your food digest after a meal, allow the wisdom of lectio to unfold within you.

Meditation: The Open Book

Sit in a comfortable seat with your spine erect. Close your eyes and welcome in a few rounds of natural breath. As you breathe, move your attention from the center of your head down your spine to the center of your chest. This is your energetic heart. Breathe here for a few moments.

Envision a book in the middle of your heart. What color is it? Are there words or images on the cover? Be as detailed or generic as you like. Now open the book. See the words scribbled across the pages. Words written on top of one another. Sentences crooked, images scrawled in the margins, everything overdone and competing for space on the page. Inhale. As you exhale, blow the words and images off the page. Watch them float into the sky and dissolve. Stay with your breath and see the open, blank pages. Sit with that for a few moments. In time, say a little prayer for guidance. Ask for a word or phrase to guide you in the days and weeks to come—one that will help you move from a place of needing to control into a partnership with God. Wait for it to arrive and then write it on the page. See it shimmer there.

When you are ready, close the book and hold it close to your heart. Return to your breath and slowly open your eyes.

Asana Practice: Forward Folds to Access Wisdom

Deep listening—to how God calls us to live and who God calls us to be— requires dedicated time to turning our attention inward. Setting aside time to practice listening on the mat builds our capacity to hear all the ways God speaks to us in daily life. As we listen to the breath and pay attention to the body's reaction to a pose or series of poses, we become accustomed to noticing our default settings. We can then ask: Is this response life-giving or life-draining?

Does pushing past pain in my shoulder result in healing or injury? Does softening the habitual tensing between my eyebrows open my receptivity?

God's call to us is always to a vital life of communion and integrity. When we listen and respond from a place of healthy yes or boundary-setting no, we step more fully onto the path of balance. Asking what season of life we are in today, and being honest about the answer, frees us to be obedient to the Grace that fills all things. In so doing, we open ourselves more fully to being the people we are called to be.

Forward folds carry an inherent energy of introspection and are a lovely companion in the practice of obedient call and response.

Balasana: Child's Pose

Begin in Child's Pose, with your feet together and your knees a comfortable hip-width distance apart or slightly wider. You may have your arms next to your body, hugging your hips, or you can extend your arms straight out in front of you, with your palms pressing down to the ground and your fingers spread wide.

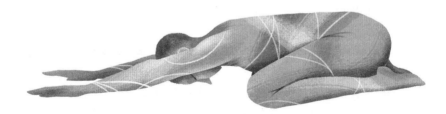

Breathe deeply. Set an intention to use this practice as a time to listen for God's call in your life. You may not hear a clear answer, but you can choose to open your ears and heart and be receptive in the days and weeks to come.

Listen to the sound of your inhale, and listen to the sound of your exhale. Feel the back of your body expand with your inhale. Become receptive to the space between your lungs, your ribs, and your vertebrae. As you exhale, relax your belly and forehead. Notice the stretch along your spine and the gentle dynamic of engagement and release in your inner thighs. Observe your body's response to this shape. If you feel you need to make any small adjustments, listen to that wisdom and honor it. See what happens when you respond to the prompting of your body and spirit.

Stay in this pose for another three to five breaths.

Marjaryasana–Bitilasana: Cat Pose–Cow Pose

Following in the wake of your breath, shift your weight forward and come to a table-top position with your knees under your hips and hands under your shoulders. Widen your feet hip-width distance apart and adjust your hands so your wrist creases are parallel to the front of your mat. Allow your fingers to gently spread. This will help soften your shoulders.

If you have knee pain, place a blanket or small towel under your knees. If you have wrist pain, place a small, rolled towel under the base of your palms to reduce the angle of bend in your wrists.

Return to an awareness of your breath. As you inhale, begin to tip your tailbone toward the backs of your knees and round your back upward. As you exhale, tip your pelvis forward to melt your belly and chest toward the floor. Lift your head as your chest expands.

Connect your movement to your breath. Listen for the moment the inhalation begins and then tip your pelvis. Notice the pause between the inhale and exhale. Wait for the next phase of the breath to begin before tipping your pelvis in the opposite direction.

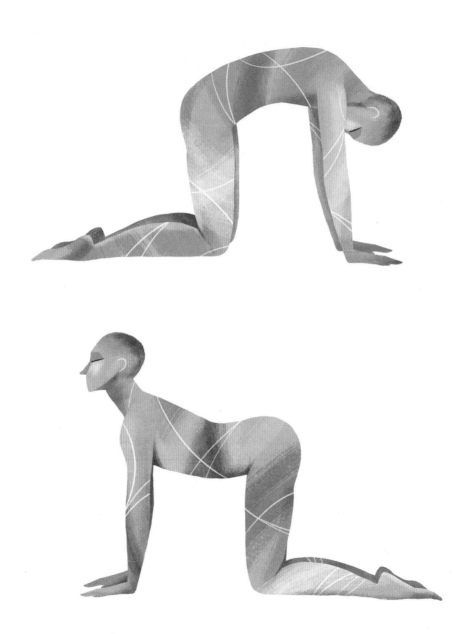

Listen, wait, respond. Engage this conversation of call and response as you round and arch your back. Press your hands and feet gently into the mat. Give a little hug of your arms toward the midline to engage your muscles. Notice how these actions affect your pose.

If it would feel good, you may make circular motions, or figure eights, with your hips. Don't overthink it. Let your body move like a wave in response to its prompting.

Continue for five to seven rounds of breath.

Adho Mukha Svanasana: Downward-Facing Dog Pose

Keeping your hands shoulder-width distance apart or perhaps slightly wider, spread your fingers like rays of the sun and press your finger pads down into the mat. Shift your hips back toward your heels and tuck your toes. Breathe here, keeping your knees on the floor, and pause.

Inhale and press your hands down into the mat as you slowly lift your hips high up to the sky. Keep your knees bent for a breath or two so that your hamstrings can engage without bracing, which will help your lower back to release. Exhale.

As you breathe, start to "walk your dog" by keeping one knee bent as you straighten the other leg, moving back and forth in concert with your breath. Avoid the tendency to rush this. Let your breath be your guide.

When you are ready, inhale and hug your arms toward the midline as you press both your legs to straight. This is Downward-Facing Dog. Notice if this creates strain or rounding in your back, however. If so, bend your knees and lift your hips a little higher.

As you exhale, keep your arms strong and soften your upper back to broaden your collarbones and open your chest, creating room for your heart to lead the way.

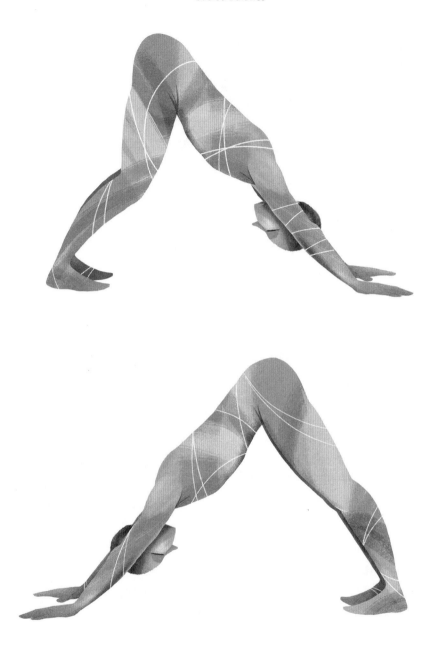

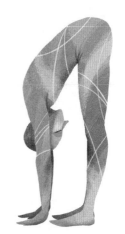

Remain in this pose for three to five breaths more if you're able; do less if your arms start to shake or you notice you can no longer hold the pose without bracing. Without judgment, listen and respond to where you are now, in a manner that promotes your health and well-being. Modify this pose using a chair or the wall, if that would be beneficial.

Uttanasana: Standing Forward Fold Pose

After a complete exhalation, walk your feet forward toward your hands to come into a Standing Forward Fold with your feet hip-width distance apart and parallel to the sides of the mat. Rest your hands on your thighs, your shins, a block, or the floor. You may bend your knees slightly or keep your legs straight.

Breathe and return to your intention. What season of life are you in? What does this season ask you to embrace or release? How can you respond?

Stay here for three to five rounds of breath.

Tadasana: Mountain Pose

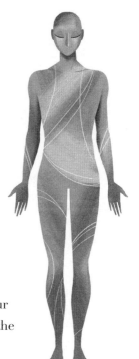

Inhale and bring your hands to your hips. Lift your shoulders so that your chest opens and your upper arms are parallel to your waist. Press your feet into the mat and firm the muscles of your legs. As you exhale, soften your effort. Inhale. Hinging from your hips, rise up to standing.

Release your hands down by your sides. Pause and stand for a few breaths. Feel the support of your feet and legs, the opening and spaciousness of your torso, and the softness of your shoulders and your face. As you continue to breathe, listen for when it is time to move to the next posture.

Prasarita Padottanasana: Wide-Legged Forward Fold Pose

Widen your stance and extend your arms out to the side. With your ankles approximately under your wrists or slightly more narrow, turn both feet to face forward. Bring your hands to your hips.

Inhale and lift your chest. Exhale and hinge forward from your hips.

You may keep your hands on your hips or bring them to the floor, a block, or the back of a chair. Look at your knees. If they are turning inward, press down through the outer edges of your feet so your arches lift and your knees can face straight forward. This will protect the joints.

Perhaps close your eyes as you breathe and release into the support of your bones. Use the time in this pose to simply focus on your breath as a way to open the ear of your heart.

Stay here for five to seven breaths.

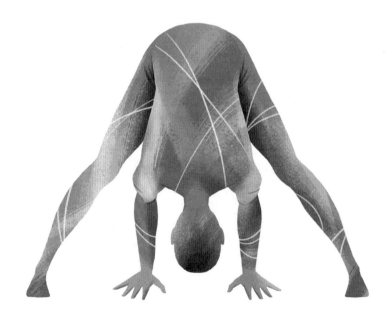

Parivrtta Janu Sirsasana:
Extended Head-to-Knee Pose with Side Bend

Come to a seated position. Extend your legs out in front of you. Inhale, then, keeping your right leg straight, bend your left knee out to the side and bring your left foot in toward your groin. Your knee will be at about a forty-five-degree angle from your hip—or less, if need be. Flex your right foot and rotate the extended leg in so the knee and toes face the sky. Exhale and shift your weight down through your left hip to settle into the support of the earth.

Place your right arm on your right thigh, the floor, or a block, then stretch your left arm up to the sky. As you reach your left arm alongside your ear, rotate your arm inward so the palm of your hand faces down. If this causes discomfort, place your left hand on your hip or lower back, palm facing up.

This pose requires deep listening to your range of motion and your current season of mobility. It is much better to back off and prop your bottom arm up than to bend too far to the side. Doing so is the intersection between humility and listening. Stay here for three to five breaths, and then repeat on the second side.

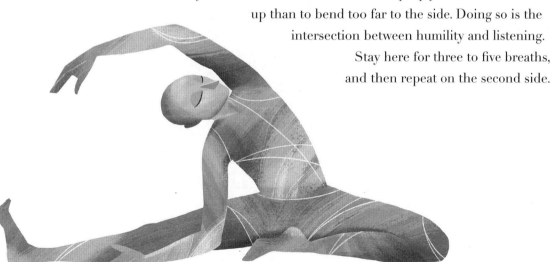

Paschimottanasana: East–West Stretch or Seated Forward Fold Pose

From the previous pose, bring your legs back to straight. Check that your knees and toes face the sky. Inhale, flex your feet, and reach your arms up to the sky. Exhale, fold from your hips, and bring your hands to your thighs or to the floor beside your hips, shins, or feet. Only go as far as you can while still breathing with ease.

Turn your attention deeply inward as you breathe and listen.

Be here for three to five breaths. When you are ready, inhale and sit back up.

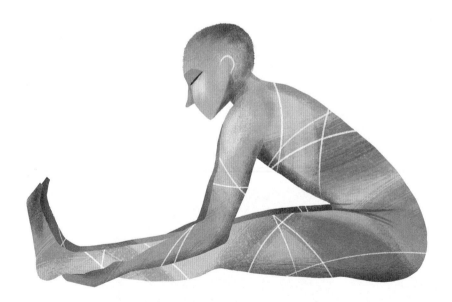

Sukhasana: Easy Pose

"Easy Pose" may sound like a misnomer for a cross-legged position that actually may be quite challenging, but it derives its name from *sukha*, meaning "ease" and *asana*, meaning "pose." Cross your legs and sit quietly, with your hands on your thighs or palms together in front of your heart. If you notice that your knees are higher than your navel, sit on blankets or blocks to encourage a release in the hamstrings and a healthy inner curve in the low back.

Close your eyes and breathe. Notice the spaciousness within yourself. Listen to the sounds around you. When you are ready, open your eyes.

Give thanks for the wisdom and guidance you receive in your practice or will receive in the day ahead.

4 Stability and Conversion
Staying and Growing

Submitting ourselves to a process of practicing

reveals secret parts of ourselves, drawing us out and

unhiding us and the holy that dwells within us.

—Jan L. Richardson

At this moment, as you read these words, you are probably sitting or lying down. You probably consider yourself being still. At rest. Doing nothing. Yet while you are just sitting there your heart is pumping blood, your breath is moving in and out, your neurons are firing, your digestive system is processing food. You are also rotating on an axis and revolving around a star at a rate of 66,000 miles an hour.

Yogis have a word for this dynamic pulsation of life: *spanda*. It refers to the contraction and expansion, the concealment and revelation, the stillness and movement. Spanda equates to the notion put forth by theoretical physics I mentioned in chapter 1, that life is both a particle and a wave.

It comforts me to know that life moves both at a great speed *and* at a long, slow pace. It comforts me to know that stillness can be found within motion and that quiet moments of reflection can be eked out of a full day. Conversely, it's comforting to know that because motion and activity are inherent parts of life, it is okay to be busy. It is okay to have a number of commitments. It is just as okay to "do" as it is to "be."

The problem emerges when our doing overrides our being, and when we are so overcommitted that we move through the day without pause or thought or breath. Similarly, a problem comes in when we "do nothing" too often, and when we grow lazy and stagnant. The yogis have words for this too. *Rajas* is the idea of fire, movement, action. Its complement is *tamas*: heaviness, slowness, inertia. The gravity of tamas, like the gravity of the earth, supports steadiness, while the intensity of rajas encourages movement. *Sattva* is the energy of clarity and purity that comes when the two are in balance.

These notions find a counterpart in two of the vows taken by Benedictine monks, nuns, and oblates: *stabilitas* (stability) and *conversatio morum* (conversion). Stabilitas, or stability, in the simplest terms, is the practice of staying put. Stability means sticking with something—a project, a location, a community— even when it gets difficult. Stability encompasses the gravity found in tamas. Conversatio morum, or conversion, is the idea of daily adjustment, growth, improvement—of failing and beginning again. Conversion requires the energy of rajas.

In Benedict's Rule, the vow of stability is the commitment monastics make to living their life in the same community, with the same people, the same personality conflicts, the same routines, in the same location day in and day out. Within that commitment is attention to a prescribed rhythm of work and prayer and dedication to a life in Christ. Benedict recognizes the tremendous challenge of this commitment and tempers it with conversion, which assumes that we will fail in our commitments, that we will fail to live in loving relationship, and that we will fail to undertake our daily tasks with joy and focus and without grumbling. A commitment to conversion reminds us that we can always begin again, and that it is through our new beginnings that we grow.

Stability outside the monastic walls doesn't necessarily look like living out our days in one location and community. What it does mean is that we commit to staying with those practices, structures, and relationships that nourish and challenge us to a life of depth and integrity anchored in love. To be clear, we are not asked to stay in relationships or situations that are toxic or abusive. Stability is not a commandment to be victimized. Rather, it is a sound call to the Ground of Being that is always the foundation and expression of love. In *Wisdom Distilled from the Daily*, Sr. Joan Chittister writes, "Stability is the one sure tool we have to be certain that the world, for us, can really become a garden to be tilled rather than a candy store to be robbed."

If humility is the groundwork for our sacred balance, stability is the root system that enables us to grow and be continually converted to new and more authentic versions of ourselves. Stability in community—whether it's a community of two or an entire cadre of persons and personalities—opens us to a larger perspective on life that encompasses the inclusive vision of Christ in the world. And we are a part of that vision.

Sticking with a community can be challenging. There are times at my church when I feel a kind of apathy, discontent, and doubt set in. The familiar and once-comforting liturgy seems stale. Nourishing relationships elude me and

I feel like an outsider or an imposter, unable to connect with others. I keep my distance to maintain a false sense of emotional security. And yet, I know that this is where I am called to grow in Grace. Here, in this community of faith, my son is being nurtured, and I am learning to be present for the community in any way I can. Stability is not just for our personal growth. We have to continually show up for others too.

Internal Stability

The technical term for a yoga pose is *asana*, which means to sit or to take a steady, comfortable seat. Originally used within the context of meditation, asana has evolved to include the yoga postures and is the suffix of the name of each pose. For example, *Trikonasana* means the seat of the *Triangle; Adho Mukha Svanasana* means the seat of Downward-Facing Dog. Adding -asana to the end of a yoga pose points us to the dynamic balance of stillness within motion and of the conversation between rajas and tamas, stability and conversion.

As with all the principles of Benedictine spirituality and yoga, there is an interior and exterior orientation. The staying power we exercise in showing up—to our prayer and meditation, our asana, our jobs, our communities—is the outer expression of interior stability strengthened by commitment. We can't cultivate our interior rootedness in love without physical practice. And our physical practice is of no use if it does not serve our inner growth.

One of the most transformational effects of inward stability is the capacity to remain with difficult thoughts and emotions without judgment or dismissal. When we come to a yoga practice, we are invited to pay attention to our body, our mind, our breath, and our emotional reactions to the postures. The same is true of meditation and contemplative prayer. Yet there's a particular potency that comes with asana. When we make a shape with the body, the muscles, organs, and energetic channels are activated in different ways. Sometimes that activation unleashes a profound joy. Sometimes it releases deep-seated anxiety or sadness or ambivalence, and we want to change shape or fidget—anything but stay with our discomfort.

But then we do. Good teachers, like a good Benedictine abbot or abbess, nudge us to stick with the pose for one breath more. They may have no idea what's going on in our internal landscape, but in that moment, they encourage us to remain steady, which breaks us open to new horizons of Grace. These shifts may be small, almost imperceptible. But change often happens in small increments that go unnoticed.

We carry these little conversions with us throughout the day. The next time we encounter a tricky relationship in our home life, our jobs, or ourselves as we spend time alone on the mat, we hear the call to pause and breathe and stay rather than run.

Stability becomes a radical affirmation. When we stay with our own emotions and allow them room to exist, we affirm the truth of our experience instead of trying to make it something other than it is. We are then better able to give room to other people to have their emotions and experience. We can stay with a friend when she is grieving. We can look her in the eyes when she is talking and think less about our response and more about what she is communicating. Through paying steady witness to our emotions, we become clear about our values and make choices with integrity.

In the gravity of tamasic stability, we kindle the fire—the rajas—necessary for transformation and conversion. Even when we feel stale, like the dormant earth in winter, there is movement and growth. Benedict calls this a growth toward a life with Christ. For the yogi, it is living into the revelation of our oneness in the body of the Divine.

In simple terms, this conversion is a movement toward being more kind and loving. Not in a passive, singsong way, but in an active call to love ourselves and our neighbor no matter how strange or different they are. The practices of stability and conversion feed Benedictine hospitality and yogic compassion, which we will explore in the following chapter.

The conversation between stability and conversion is a lived journey into sacred balance. We seek out habits, routines, relationships, and attitudes that root us in love, while remaining open to the often surprising and perhaps uncomfortable ways we are nudged again and again toward the outer expression of that love.

In *Always We Begin Again: The Benedictine Way of Living*, John McQuistin II writes: "Each good action we perform is like a blow from a sculptor's chisel, cutting away the dross, and shaping the ideal form hidden within the stone. Each step we take away from hidden dependence on material possessions is like a day of training for an athlete, strengthening ourselves into the fit and healthy persons we were designed to be. It is the small, daily brush strokes that create the painting, no matter how large the canvas."

It is the small, daily practices to which we commit—the moments and people we choose to stay with rather than abandon, the asanas we hold, and the prayer we make space for—that keep us ever steady in growth toward a more full, complete expression of ourselves within a God of love.

Statio: Stillpoint between Steadiness and Motion

In the days before my son was born, my centering routine looked very different than it does today. I would rise early, read a daily meditation for lectio divina, journal, spend an hour or so in asana, and then move about my day. I'd stop working around four o'clock in the afternoon, walk the dog, meditate for thirty minutes, and then make dinner.

Now I am a single mom who works full time outside the home. I don't have long, open spaces of time to devote to extended practice. What I do have is a commitment to what is essential for keeping me oriented toward a life of wellness, love, and integrity. I still rise early to practice asana and sit in prayer. My lectio practice is haphazard, though I always create just a few minutes to read something of Spirit. Sometimes I journal. Sometimes I meditate. Though the dog died in the intervening years, I still do my best to walk outside for at least a few minutes each day to breathe fresh air and reorient my mind and spirit. The daily and seasonal rhythms we'll explore in chapters 6 and 7 guide my day. My steadfast commitment to these simple practices brings an equanimity to my life that I miss during periods in which I give them up to busyness and overexertion. Like a tree firmly planted in the earth, they grant me the steadiness out of which to grow.

Because balance is a dynamic conversation between stability and movement, our practices need to evolve and adapt to our life's circumstance. Through humility and the deep listening of obedience, we begin to recognize where and how we remain rooted. Yet there is one practice we can wholeheartedly embrace, regardless of the season and circumstances of life, and that is *statio*.

Statio is the monastic practice of pausing at the end of one task, before beginning another. It's as simple and forgettable as that. In pausing, we open the smallest of spaces within for the largesse of Presence to be revealed. In that holy pause, we reconnect with our roots, which extend into the Ground of Being. In that space, we can grow alongside the Grace that carries us forward.

It is so easy just to move from one activity or task to the next, without taking the time to slow down for a moment and pay attention to where we are and what we are doing. I am guilty of this. It helps to begin by attaching an intentional statio to a repetitive task. Pause before making a phone call or sending an email.

Pause and breathe for a few minutes in the car before going to work or picking up your child from school. Pause before a meal and give thanks for the food you are to receive and the many hands that brought it to your table.

In our asana, we cultivate our capacity for statio by linking movement with breath. We pause, breathe, and then move. When we hold a pose and focus on the rhythms of breath, we invite ourselves to settle into the pause between inhale and exhale, exhale and inhale. Through statio, we tap into the dynamic stillpoint between steadiness and motion, stability and conversion, rajas and tamas.

Statio is also crucial in our efforts to be loving members of any community. We can pause before speaking. We can make a habit of stopping the busywork and engaging with our family, colleagues, and children. We can take a deep breath and read the news so we become aware of the world around us and pray for how we may respond to the needs of our society. We can look away from our screens and up at the sky to marvel at God's creation. Each pause, then, becomes an acceptance of the invitation to a life growing in Grace.

Questions for Reflection

- What are the practices in your life that keep you steady? A daily devotion, a walk, a mass, a meditation, a yoga practice, a prayer? Pick one or two and commit to using them each day for one week.

- How do you practice the vow of stability in community?

- What growth have you experienced when you've stayed put, whether emotionally, physically, or spiritually?

- When can you practice statio—intentional pause— throughout your day?

Wellness Practice: Drink Hot Water

The practice of drinking hot water first thing in the morning and throughout the day can have a profound effect on our ability to stay balanced and steady. Hot water has a grounding, tamasic effect while also invigorating the rajas of digestion. A student called it a "loving hug for your insides." Drinking hot water, while it may seem small and inconsequential, invites a slowness, a holy pause.

As soon as possible after getting out of bed, boil some water and drink two to three cups hot. You may mix in a little room-temperature water if you prefer, or you may also choose to add a slice of lemon for extra flavor.

Drink your hot water before drinking any coffee or tea and preferably before any food. Many people have found that having hot water before coffee reduces or delays their need for caffeine. If possible, sip your hot water throughout the day. When you feel like snacking, try a little hot water first and see if that takes the emotional edge off the need for extra food. Sometimes it will, sometimes it won't.

As you sip your hot water, read a daily devotion or look out the window and watch the natural world around you: the steadiness of trees, the vastness of sky, a potted plant, a sleeping pet. Notice how your nervous system responds to this moment of pause and reflection. Watch how the hot water and gentle meditation slows you down just enough to experience stillness within movement.

Meditation: The Willow Tree

When you look at a picture of the human nervous system, the nerves of the legs extend downward like tree roots and those of the arms extend out like the soft branches of the willow tree. It's quite beautiful. Willow trees, while they may appear delicate at first, are strong and resilient because their form has a balance of steadiness and the ability to move and adapt to the wind and weather. We will use this imagery—of the body having roots and branches like the willow tree— to promote our connection to stability and growth.

Sit comfortably in a chair or on the floor. You might even choose to do this meditation outside and sit directly on the earth.

Close your eyes and enjoy a few rounds of deep breathing. When you are ready, begin to soften into a more relaxed rhythm of inhalation and exhalation. As you breathe, turn your attention inward and drop your awareness from the center of your head, down your spine, through your heart, and deep into the base of your seat. Feel the chair, the floor, or the earth beneath you. Imagine roots reaching down through your spine and tailbone and burrowing deep into the warmth and nourishing darkness of the earth. Locate all the meeting points of your body and the floor, and imagine extending roots down from them as well.

Then begin to extend your attention back up through the trunk of your body. Feel yourself growing tall, reaching up to the sky. Imagine the long, soft branches of a willow tree cascading up and out from your center. Your core remains steady and strong even as the branches sway and dance in the wind. You create a grove of shade, a center of solace, as you welcome members of your community to rest under your limbs.

Stay here for some time, feeling your roots support you as you grow and sway and embrace.

When you are ready, give thanks for the community you welcomed into your presence. Offer gratitude for the earth that supports you and the winds that move you. Return your attention to your body. Breathe well, and open your eyes.

Asana Practice: Standing Poses for Grounding and Mobility

Standing poses can ground the energy of the body and leave us feeling strong, capable, and ready to meet the demands of the day. An essential principle in any yoga posture is "root to rise." After we pause, breathe, and welcome in a bigger energy, we feel into the foundation of a pose—the tactile sensation of the feet and hands on the mat, the strength and support of the arms and legs. Next we draw energy from the foundation up, to our center of gravity, like a tree drinking in nourishment from the earth. This center of gravity is the core of the pelvis in standing and seated postures, for example, and the back of the heart in Downward-Facing Dog. From the center of gravity we extend energy back out the core lines of the body to the foundation. In a standing pose, this has the effect of creating strength in the legs and dynamic stability in the core and upper body that promotes greater mobility and freedom of breath. Without this stable foundation, the rest of the pose becomes disconnected from the core. If that happens, we risk a sense of disintegration and perhaps injury as we try to push too far.

Standing poses are some of the first taught to beginners because they strengthen the legs and hips while also improving range of movement. They can be done in the middle of the room, or near a wall or chair for balance. If you have the benefit of practicing your asana with a friend, try facing each other so that you can support each other's growth.

In each pose, watch the steadiness of your body coupled with the movement of your inhale and exhale, the beating of your heart, and the dynamic of rooting down to rise up to the sky. Observe your physical, mental, and emotional reactions to each pose. Without judgment, allow yourself to stay

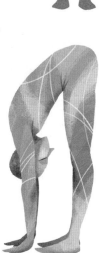

with the experience of letting breath, thoughts, emotions, and physical sensations rise and fall on their own. Practice pausing before you move to the next pose.

Tadasana: Mountain Pose

Stand with your feet hip-width distance apart and parallel. Let your arms hang down by your sides. Breathe gently in and out through your nose, sending your breath deep into your lungs. Rock forward and backward on your feet, and then come to rest. Like a tree pulling nutrients from the earth, inhale and draw strength from your feet up through your legs and spine and raise your arms overhead. Exhale and lower them down to your sides. Staying strong and steady in your legs, lift your arms out and overhead several times.

When you are ready, exhale and bring your hands to your hips.

Uttanasana: Standing Forward Fold Pose

With your hands on your hips, inhale and hinge forward. Bring your hands to touch something tangible—the floor, your legs, the back of a chair, a block—to make a steady connection from the periphery of your body to something unwavering. Exhale and soften your belly and shoulders.

Stay here for a few breaths, then bring your hands to your hips and rise back up to standing.

Virabhadrasana II: Warrior II Pose

Raise your arms out to the side and separate your feet so they are approximately under your wrists. Rotate your right leg out so the toes face the top of your mat. Keeping your arms outstretched, turn your head to look out past your right hand. Inhale and bend your right knee toward ninety

degrees, aligning your knee over your ankle. As you breathe, continue the dynamic of drawing strength and steadiness from your feet up to your pelvis and rooting back down to cultivate stability. Notice how this supports a natural buoyancy in your upper body.

Stay here for three to five breaths, then repeat in the other direction with your left foot forward.

Utthita Parsvakonasana: Extended Side Angle Pose

Setting up in the same wide stance you used for the previous pose, rotate your right leg out and bend your right knee toward ninety degrees. Inhale and lower your right forearm to your right thigh, and stretch your left arm up to the sky. Stretch from your pelvis down through the bones of your back leg, rooting into the support of the ground. Draw strength back up through your legs and reach through the sides of your waistline up to your top fingers. If you'd like, internally rotate your top arm so the pinky finger faces the floor and sweep the arm alongside your ear.

Stay here for three to five breaths. Inhale, exhale, and stretch back down through your left leg and foot and rise back up through your torso. Rotate your right leg in and your left leg out to switch the direction and repeat on the second side.

Optional Flow: Warrior II to Extended Side Angle Pose

If you'd like to bring a little fluid movement to your practice, you can flow between Warrior II and Extended Side Angle poses for a few breaths.

Return to Warrior II.
Inhale. Exhale and lower

your front forearm to your thigh and extend your back arm up. Breathe. Draw in to your core. Inhale and extend down through your back foot as you lift your torso and return to Warrior II. Repeat the flow between these poses several times, coordinating the movement with the breath. Notice how staying steady through your legs and feet makes the movement of the upper body integrated.

Trikonasana: Triangle Pose

Maintain your wide stance. Inhale and turn your right leg out. Exhale. Bring your hands to your hips. Inhale and lift your chest. Exhale and hinge from your hips to tip to the right. Lower your right hand along your inner thigh, calf, or to the floor or a block behind your right foot. Stretch your left arm to the sky. It is important to keep your head in line with your pelvis and the side of your body parallel to the floor. If you feel you are tipping or rounding forward, bring your bottom hand higher up your leg. With every inhale, draw steadiness from your feet and arms into your pelvis. With every exhale, root from your pelvis back down through your legs to your feet and extend up through your top arm to the sky.

Stay in this pose for three to five breaths. Root down through your back leg, inhale, and lift your torso. Pause, then repeat on the second side.

Vrksasana: Tree Pose

Tree Pose is a balance posture. You may use one hand on a chair or the wall for support if you need it. Stand on your right leg and bring your left foot to your ankle, your calf, or your upper inner thigh. Be sure that your foot is well above or below your knee so there is no pressure on the knee joint. With one or both hands on your hips, inhale to create space. Exhale to soften. With your next inhalation, press your standing leg and lifted foot together so that you draw stability in to your core. With your exhale, extend steady energy from your pelvis down through your standing leg and reach your arms up to the sky.

You may notice that your standing foot wavers. That's okay. Remember: balance is a dynamic of steadiness and motion. Like a tree swaying in the wind, you can allow your muscles to be firm even while you allow for gentle movement. Let your body respond to the rise and fall of your breath.

Breathe here for three to five rounds of breath. Place your left foot back on the floor and stand in Mountain Pose for one breath before moving to the second side. When you've completed your final exhale on the second side, place your foot back on the ground.

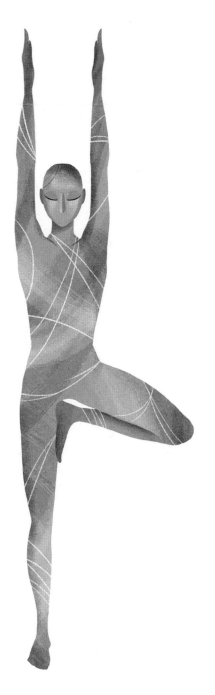

Tadasana: Mountain Pose

Stand in Mountain Pose for a few breaths to close your
practice. Keeping your feet hip-width distance apart
and parallel, bring your hands together in front of
your heart. Close your eyes and observe your
steadiness. Feel the free movement of your
breath within your stable body.

Say a prayer or offering of thanks.

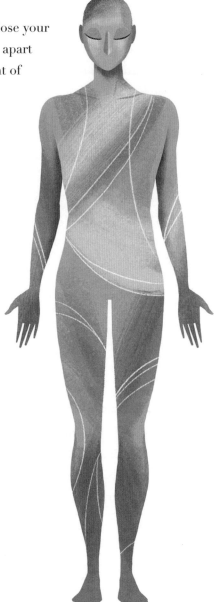

5 Hospitality
Welcoming Companions

Will you seek and serve Christ in all persons, loving your neighbor as yourself? . . . Will you strive for justice and peace among all people, and respect the dignity of every human being?

—Baptismal Covenant, *Book of Common Prayer*

Namaste. You've probably heard this word or seen it on T-shirts, email signatures, or yoga studios. It is a common greeting, and often offered as a blessing at the end of a yoga class.

Nama means "bow," *as* means "I," and *te* means "you," so the basic translation is "I bow to you." The beauty of the Sanskrit language is that words may have deeper meanings and associations that refer more to concepts than to a singular word or phrase when translated to English. Namaste is a simple greeting that confers respect. Further, this greeting may connote an attitude that recognizes our shared indwelling Divine Consciousness. Christians might interpret this to mean a recognition of the indwelling Christ in all of us. From this deeper level, to offer a namaste is to say that the place within me where Divine Love dwells bows to the same place of Divine Love in you. Namaste is a choice to affirm the dignity and worth of all beings, including ourselves. The Tantra lineage—a non-dual branch of yoga philosophy focusing on experience of the Divine—teaches that the universe is all one Divine Consciousness longing to experience itself in many forms. Taken in this context, namaste is a greeting that upholds our oneness *and* celebrates what makes us unique.

Benedict's Rule does just that. In the chapters on provision in the Rule, each monk is given exactly what he needs to live his life with enough worldly goods—clothing, bedding, food, and drink—to be comfortable and prevent grumbling. Each member of the community is given jobs that develop or use their strengths. While cultivating individual gifts, monastics are also tasked with a deep, heartfelt recognition that we all dwell in the one heart of Christ. Our differences and similarities are part of the great Communion.

In the Benedictine Way, special attention is to be given to guests. Everyone is welcome at the monastery regardless of age, class, wealth, gender, or race: "All guests who present themselves are to be welcomed as Christ, who said: 'I was a stranger and you welcomed me'" (Rule 53, Matthew 25:35). Guests are to be given the same provision as the monks and are to be welcomed into the community and invited to prayer. "Once the guests have been announced, the prioress or abbot and the community are to meet them with all the courtesy of love." (Rule 53). More than basic necessities, guests are to be given warmth, acceptance, enjoyment, and celebration. Special attention is to be given to the poor, because culture automatically affords more respect to the rich.

In the aftermath of the Roman Empire, when Benedict wrote his Rule, travel was dangerous and monasteries became safe havens for those on a journey. Receiving guests was a natural occurrence in the life of the monks. While a guest may show up unannounced at any hour and be given proper attention, their presence was not to disturb the rhythms of work and prayer that make up communal life. This boundary-setting by the community both upholds self-care and fosters the capacity to wholeheartedly extend lovingkindness to others.

Like namaste—and like humility, obedience, stability, and conversion— hospitality has both an interior and exterior orientation. How often do we find it easier to offer a warm welcome to others than to extend the same kindness to ourselves? It is all too easy to succumb to self-flagellation for our fears, foibles, mistakes, and eccentricities. We are too hard on ourselves. We reject and push away those thoughts and emotions we view as negative, berating their very existence. What if, instead of habitually treating ourselves so harshly, we practiced radical hospitality by welcoming and giving space at the table for all parts of ourselves? How much more accepting of others would we be if we could first accept ourselves?

As my own worst critic, I understand how lofty this is. Yet through my commitment to hospitality, I do what I can to practice loving reception for myself by cultivating what can be called an "inner witness." An inner witness is a character of loving detachment—an observer within the self that watches the rise and fall of emotions, the actions and reactions, without judgment. Seeing these emotions for what they are—a part of being human—the inner witness can help us reframe feelings we've judged to be negative. By taking the stance of the inner witness, I am able to give space for all parts of myself to exist, especially those parts that cause discomfort.

Here is where stability and hospitality intersect. By living into the vow of stability, I stick with an emotion, giving it time to develop and dissipate, which it will. We can think of emotions as e-motions: energy in motion. The body has a physical reaction to each emotion. Attuning to the tensing and gripping and opening of our bodies, we begin to recognize the limited life cycle of an emotion. No one emotion—no one discomfort—lasts forever, even when it feels prolonged for days, weeks, months, or years. Eventually something will shift. Our capacity for balance is directly related to our capacity to embrace the fluctuations of our inner and outer worlds.

The yogic values of *karuna* and *daya* are those of compassion. Karuna refers to feelings of warmth, empathy, and tenderness. The tantric scholar and professor William K. Mahony posits that the related concept of daya is the active component of karuna. The *da* in daya is based on the verb *dā*, which means "to give." So daya is a quality of generosity of spirit. Harkening back to the full expression of Benedictine hospitality, the yogi doesn't just feel warmth, doesn't just offer provisions, but does so with a generous spirt. Outward actions spring from inner love and welcoming. In his wonderful book *Exquisite Love: Heart-Centered Reflections on the Nārada Bhakti Sūtra*, Mahony writes: "In the yogic context, this compassionate giving also involves the act of dwelling in the true Self, Ātman—the same Self that resides within the other, too. Charitable communion with the Self is the immersion into and participation in the Divine Presence in all beings. Compassionate love thus recognizes and honors the Self—both in the being of the other *and* in one's own being."

Benedictine hospitality, yogic compassion, and generosity are all key elements on the path of sacred balance. As I write this, my five-year-old is going through a phase of having a difficult time going to bed at night. At the end of a long day, I am too easily short with him as I struggle to navigate the fine line between helping him manage his fears and succumbing to what sometimes feels like manipulation to sleep in my bed. It occurs to me that my harsh voice and clear frustration are not extending hospitality to every part of him. When I use my inner witness to see that my anger is a manifestation of a deeper fear—that I'm not doing this parenting thing right because he's not doing exactly what I want him to do—I can more easily take a step back and meet him where he is with active compassion. In doing this, I don't discount or push away my own fear and insecurity; I give it room to exist without letting it dictate my actions. By giving myself room to exist, I am able to be a more compassionate presence for my son.

As we seek a more balanced lifestyle, it is helpful to locate those circumstances and emotions that throw us off center. Rather than succumb to the temptation of believing that the spiritual life is all peace and loveliness, we can remember that it's the totality of our experience, and how we respond to it, that counts.

Giving Welcome

My son's godmother, who is a dear friend, came over for lunch one day. I rushed home from work to cook us a simple meal of scrambled eggs and summer vegetables, and she brought extra goodies to share. As we were eating and chatting, I noticed that there were crumbs on the table, because the night before I had been tired and had forgotten to wipe it down after dinner. Acting on reflex, I blurted out an embarrassed apology for the state of my table.

"It's okay," she replied. "I was just thinking how nice it is to know I'm not the only one whose house is a little messy."

There is a pervasive cultural undercurrent that in order to truly receive guests in our home, we must have the place looking spotless. Anything less is seen as a sign of disrespect. To be sure, we want to greet those who enter our homes with a reasonable degree of cleanliness, but there is no inherent value in perfection. When I visit friends—especially those with young children—toys on the floor, school papers piled on the counters, and the hum of the dishwasher in the background provide more comfort to me than a magazine-worthy home would. It is the warmth of spirit, not the level of tidiness, that makes a home inviting.

Warmth of spirit and the capacity to extend oneself, messiness and all, is what allows us to offer radical hospitality to those we meet. When we do the work to humbly accept ourselves as we are and make space for the parts of ourselves we'd rather not entertain, it becomes much easier to welcome others, whether that welcome is into our homes, our churches, our yoga studios, or our countries.

Benedict echoes Jesus's teaching to welcome all and, in doing so, to affirm the Christ in each and every person we meet. Like the rest of the spiritual life, this is not easy. There are simply going to be people we don't like, people who feel unsafe, and relationships that become toxic and need to change. And that's okay. Healthy boundaries are important. But what Jesus, Benedict, and the yogis call us to do is pause and move beyond our first impulse to reject and judge. We are called to welcome into community the stranger, the refugee, and the people who don't look like us into community. We can offer hospitality by returning to the stance of namaste and trying, at least for a moment, to see the indwelling Grace in all people. On behalf of people we see as causing great harm to us or to others, we can offer prayers: that we may be open to the love of God, that we can extend that love to them in whatever way we can, that they might be transformed by love. And then we translate that love into action, whether on an individual, societal, or global level.

In *Traveling Mercies: Some Thoughts on Faith*, Anne Lamott writes that Grace "meets us where we are but does not leave us where it found us." When we offer sincere hospitality to others and give them a seat at the table—whether it's in our homes, in traffic, in line at the supermarket, or in our chosen communities—we become forces of Grace able to meet people where they are, give them warmth, and send them away with some inkling of the comfort of God. In doing so, we bring into balance the hospitality we long for ourselves with the hospitality longed for by the world. We recognize our interdependence and connect more deeply with creation from a place of love.

Questions for Reflection

- How do you practice hospitality to yourself and others?
- What parts of yourself do you tend to push away?
- Can you stay with the discomfort you feel, offering a loving witness to its existence?
- Who do you welcome?
- Who do you exclude? Why? How could you make space for them in your heart and possibly your life?
- When someone interrupts your work or your daily plans, how can you show more lovingkindness while still upholding your boundaries?

Wellness Practice: Do Oil Massage

The practice of *abhyanga*—oil massage—is a deep and healing way to care for your body and extend generous welcome and acceptance to yourself.

The skin is the largest organ in the body. It is one of the primary organs for processing and eliminating toxins. The skin is exposed to a significant amount of pollution and should thus be cared for as holistically as possible. When the skin gets too dry, from the Ayurvedic perspective, we increase our capacity for disease because the lymphatic system—which is responsible for collecting and removing waste from the body—gets clogged and grows stagnant. Providing healthy moisture to the skin stimulates optimal lymphatic flow.

Oil massage has a host of benefits, including nourishing and rejuvenating the mind and body, enhancing the complexion, soothing the nervous system, enhancing circulation, promoting sleep and relieving fatigue, building stamina, releasing stress, awakening the senses, recovering from muscle fatigue, and supporting digestion, blood pressure, and organ communication. When we're feeling ungrounded, overwhelmed, or keyed up, oil massage can calm us down. When we're feeling lethargic or sluggish, oil massage—or its partner *garshana*, or dry brushing—provides gentle stimulation. Garshana has similar benefits of nourishing the body, calming the nervous system, and stimulating lymphatic flow and is a good option if you tend to have oily skin.

Incorporating abhyanga or garshana into your daily routine can create an environment in your body that welcomes whatever comes your way—toxic or beneficial—and processes it accordingly. Going further, the very act of massaging your body forces you to meet yourself where you are and affords an opportunity to extend some lovingkindness to others. Offering abhyanga in a safe way to a friend or loved one is a beautiful opportunity to extend hospitality and welcoming. Once a week or so, after my son's bath, he puts on his pajama shorts and lets me rub shea butter into his skin. He sighs with delight and relaxes. Appropriate touch can be a powerful communicator of love.

Choose oils that are pure, such as coconut, sesame, or almond. If you tend to have oily skin, you may opt for dry brushing instead, using gloves, a soft brush, or just your hands. Oils or dry brushing are best, but a thick butter, such as shea, works as well. Be sure that whatever you use has few to no additives, so avoid commercial lotions. We want to saturate the skin with nourishment, not bombard it with more than can be easily processed. You may also experiment with adding essential oils to further enhance the experience.

Technique

Traditionally, abhyanga is done fifteen to twenty minutes or so before a bath so the oil has a chance to soak deep into the skin. Not many of us, myself included, have that kind of time, however, so a more realistic method is to do abhyanga before or just after getting out of the shower.

Abhyanga is also optimal when done with warm oil. You can warm the oil by placing the bottle in a cup or bowl of hot water prior to use. This is the traditional method and feels delightful, but it is not essential.

Start with your scalp, if you don't mind oil in your hair; if you do, skip it. Rub oil with love and vigor into your skin. Use long strokes on the limbs and circular movements on the joints. Pay special attention to the parts you tend to criticize. The same is true for dry brushing.

There's no need to overthink this! Give yourself the oil massage in a spirit of generosity. Notice how it affects the quality not just of your skin but of your mind and emotions as well. Abhyanga and dry brushing are incredibly balancing. This is also a great practice to teach children.

Meditation: Lovingkindness

This meditation can increase our compassion for ourselves and one another. It is adapted from the Buddhist compassion, or lovingkindness, meditation as outlined in *The Book of Joy* by His Holiness the Dalai Lama, Archbishop Desmond Tutu, and Douglas Abrams. Practicing this meditation creates space within our hearts to recognize the suffering and joy of other people and thus makes us more aware of and responsive to the needs of others. In doing so, hospitality becomes more than just welcoming people into our homes and sphere of life but about radically affirming our shared human family.

The meditation moves through several stages, beginning with a loved one, ourselves, a community, a difficult person or group of persons, and a recognition of all beings on the planet. When we acknowledge another person's suffering—particularly the suffering of someone with whom we disagree—we teach ourselves to welcome people where they are and let go of labels that make them easier to dismiss.

Begin by finding a comfortable seated posture. Close your eyes and breathe deeply to draw your attention inward. When you feel ready, release back into a natural rhythm of breath.

Stage One: Hospitality and Compassion for a Loved One

1. Call to mind the image of a loved one. It could be a person or a beloved pet. Saturate your awareness with their presence. Become attentive to the sensations in your body: your face, your neck, your chest, your belly, your heart. Notice what your love for this person or pet feels like on an energetic and visceral level. Keeping this sensory awareness, hold the image of your loved one in mind and offer them the following blessing:

May you be safe and free from suffering,

May you be healthy and strong,

May you be happy,

May you live with peace and joy.

2. As you breathe, imagine a warm light from your heart wrapping your loved one in care and tenderness.

3. Celebrate your loved one's happiness.

4. Recall a moment or situation when your loved one had a difficult time, was ill, or perhaps did something you did not like. Notice what it feels like to physically and energetically connect with their pain. How does your heart feel? Your stomach? Your face? How did you respond in that situation?

5. Once again offer them the blessing.

6. Extend love from your heart and wrap them in your care.

Stage Two: Hospitality and Compassion for Self

1. Keeping the feeling of tenderness and kindness you hold for your loved one, visualize yourself. Perhaps this is an image of yourself smiling. Or consider a time when you had difficulty, whether it was a circumstance or self-imposed judgment.

2. See yourself wrapped in a warm glow of light and love emanating from your own heart as you offer the blessing:

May I be safe and free from suffering,

May I be healthy and strong,

May I be happy,

May I live with peace and joy.

3. If it is difficult to extend this radical hospitality to yourself, consider a time when you received a warm welcome or were met with care when you were experiencing pain. Let that feeling and memory be your guide as you offer the blessing.

Stage Three: Hospitality and Compassion for Community

1. Visualize a community you wish to support. This could be members of your biological or chosen family, a church group, children who are hungry, people who are marginalized, or individuals who are abused or violated.

2. Feel their joy or pain and notice what happens in your body. Does your heart rejoice or ache? Do you cry out for love?

3. Come back to the visceral feelings of compassion and tenderness you held for your loved one and extend that from your heart, wrapping this community in welcoming love as you offer the blessing:

May they be safe and free from suffering,

May they be healthy and strong,

May they be happy,

May they live with joy and peace.

4. Hold them in your heart for some time.

Stage Four: Hospitality and Compassion for Those We Would Rather Exclude

1. Return to the image of your beloved and the feelings of expansive kindness and love you hold for that person or pet. Feel it in your body, mind, and heart.

2. Now call to mind a person or group of persons you have difficulty with. This could be someone in your immediate family or a person or group of persons on a global scale with whom you profoundly disagree or whom you blame for the suffering of others. This can be the most difficult and ultimately transformative stage of the meditation, because it challenges us to follow Jesus's teaching to love all, even those we find most unlovable.

3. Notice how your body feels. What happens to the physical sensations of love? Does your jaw tense? Do your eyes narrow? Do you experience anger? That's okay. Feel what you feel.

4. If you are able, offer that person or group of persons the same warmth you offered to others thus far. If you are unable to do so, ask that God may extend the love you find challenging and that you may one day love as well.

5. With or without the physical and energic sensation of love and kindness, remember that this this person or group of persons experiences and perhaps acts from their own pain and suffering. Notice how that recognition affects your feelings.

6. With sincerity offer them the blessing:

May you be safe and free from suffering,

May you be healthy and strong,

May you be happy,

May you live with peace and joy.

7. Breathe and stay with this for a few moments.

Stage Five: Hospitality and Compassion for All Beings

1. Call to mind the vision of our entire human family. Recognize that all beings long to experience love and kindness and be free from suffering and rejection.

2. Extend warmth and love from your heart center to our shared community and repeat the blessing:

May we be safe and free from suffering,

May we be healthy and strong,

May we be happy,

May we live with peace and joy.

3. Breathe and settle into this expansive love and radical hospitality emanating from the core of your heart, recognizing that as you do so, you are acting as a vehicle for God's grace in the world.

These stages are guidelines for practice. Sometimes you may wish to focus the entirety of your lovingkindness meditation on individuals you love and care for. You may also choose to focus on groups of people, or even sit entirely with the call to extend radical hospitality to those you find difficult to love. Whatever way you choose to do this practice, I suggest starting from an awareness of and blessing for a particular loved one. That way you place yourself within a pattern of energetic and physical compassion, which will guide and imprint the rest of your meditation.

Asana Practice: Gentle Backbends to Open the Chest and Heart

Backbends are often considered the most transformational class of yoga postures. They expand the lungs for better breathing, bring a supple strength to the core muscles of the torso, invigorate the nervous system, and open and support the energetic heart located in the center of the chest. So often we hunch our upper backs, round our shoulders forward, and compress our chests. This can happen as a result of close-up work on a computer, manual labor that requires stooping, or a pernicious feeling of overwhelm.

With countless demands on our time and attention, a barrage of emotional triggers, and the chaotic state of global affairs, many of us look as though we carry the weight of the world on our shoulders. To guard against this endless onslaught, we may unconsciously close ourselves off physically, emotionally, and spirituality.

Both Benedict and the practice of yoga call us to a posture of open-heartedness, which welcomes ourselves and others with compassion. Back-bending is a powerful way to cultivate this internal and external orientation of hospitality.

The poses in this sequence are gentle and can be done by almost anyone. Pay careful attention to the alignment instructions, however, particularly if you have any structural issues in your spine such as herniated or compressed discs. If you have questions or concerns, consult your health-care professional before you begin.

Marjaryasana–Bitilasana: Cat Pose–Cow Pose

Come to a table-top position with your knees under your hips and hands under your shoulders. Widen your feet hip-width distance apart and rotate your wrists so their creases are parallel to the front of your mat. Allow your fingers to gently spread. This will help soften your shoulders.

If you have knee pain, place a blanket or small towel under your knees. If you have wrist pain, place a small, rolled towel under the base of your palms to reduce the angle of bend in your wrists.

Bring awareness to your breath. As you inhale, begin to tip your tailbone toward the backs of your knees and round your back upward. Let your head release downward. This is Cat Pose. As you exhale, tip your pelvis forward to melt your belly and chest toward to the floor. Lift your head as your chest expands. This is Cow Pose.

Continue to flow between arching and releasing your back. Let each movement follow in the wake of your breath. Feel the expanse of your back as you round the spine, and feel the softening of your belly as you melt. Notice the

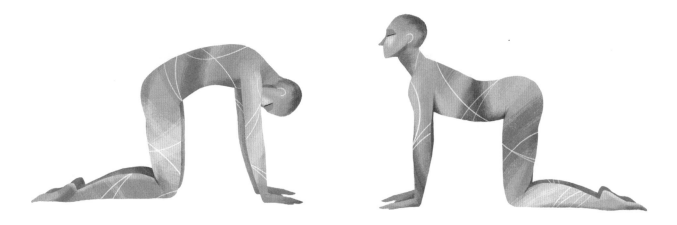

dynamic relationship between broadening your back as you round and expanding your chest and collarbones as you melt your belly toward the floor.

With each inhale, welcome in the sensation of your body. Welcome in your experience. With each exhale, let go of the need to judge or control it.

Move through this flow between poses for several rounds of breath, and then return to a neutral spine.

Adho Mukha Svanasana: Downward-Facing Dog Pose

Shift your hips back to your heels. Tuck your toes and reach your arms forward, keeping hands shoulder-width distance apart. Breathe.

Inhale and press your inner and outer hands and finger pads into the mat to evenly engage the muscles of your arms. Exhale and settle in to your physical experience.

On your next inhale, lift your knees off the floor and reach your hips to the sky. If your lower back rounds or you feel strain in your back or hamstrings, keep your knees bent. Otherwise you may press your legs to straight. Exhale.

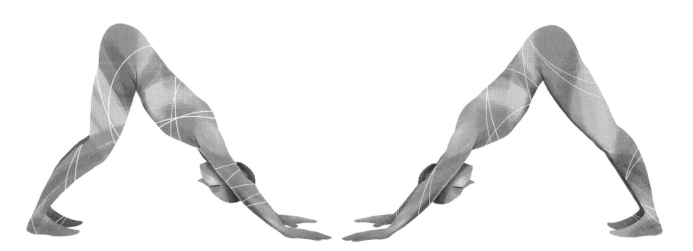

As you inhale, gather support up from your hands, through the bones of your arms, and into the back of your energetic heart, located between your shoulder blades. Exhale and soften your heart space.

Stay in Downward-Facing Dog for three to five breaths. If you can only do one breath, wonderful. If you are unable to support yourself, modify with Child's Pose. Allow each breath to be an opportunity to welcome yourself exactly as you are in this moment. Give room for the joy and frustration, the confusion and clarity, the anxiety and peace. Gather it all in your heart, then release it back down through your hands and feet into the support of a loving Power, which is greater than yourself.

Tadasana: Mountain Pose

From Downward-Facing Dog, inhale and step your feet between your hands. Pause in *Uttanasana*, Standing Forward Fold. Exhale. Inhale and rise up to standing.

Stand in Mountain Pose for a few breaths. Bring your attention to your heart space, located in the center of your chest between your breastbone and shoulder blades. You may wish to bring one hand on top of the other over your heart and breathe here. How does your heart feel? Is it constricted? Open? Wounded? Trusting? What or whom can you welcome into your life today?

Uttanasana with Heart Opening: Standing Forward Fold with Hands Clasped Pose

Behind your back, interlace your fingers and clasp your hands. Place your thumbs to your sacrum—the triangular bone at the base of your spine—to stay connected to all parts of your interior and exterior experience.

Inhale and lift up through the sides of your waistline. Exhale and gently roll your shoulders back so that the bases of your shoulder blades hug toward each other.

Keeping your hands clasped and your elbows bent, inhale, exhale, and fold forward from your hips. Bend your knees, if that feels comfortable. You may keep your hands touching your sacrum or stretch them overhead, allowing gravity to help you release.

As you breathe here for three to five breaths, continue to lift your shoulders up so your chest and collarbones broaden. Cultivate the capacity to meet yourself and the world with an open heart, supported by the Divine.

When you are ready, release the clasp of your hands and return to standing position.

Bhujangasana: Cobra Pose

Lie down on your belly. With your hands on the floor alongside your chest, welcome in a full breath as you soften your abdomen. Inhale and press the tops of your feet down to root into a strong foundation. Lift your shoulders toward the center of your back. Exhale and soften through your chest.

Keeping your shoulders back, press your hands down as you inhale and lift your belly, chest, and torso off the mat. Exhale.

Depending on your comfort level, you may simply lift your chest an inch or so off the mat for what is called Baby Cobra. Do what feels right for your body. This is our first back bend. If you experience pain or pinching in your lower back, keep the lift in your chest small and your belly on the floor to practice a modified version of this pose.

There is a tendency to round the shoulders forward or pull them up toward the ears. As you breathe, consciously bring your shoulders back and softly down away from your ears so that your chest opens and you cultivate space for a bigger breath—a breath that can welcome and embrace all those you will meet today. If doing this is difficult with your belly and chest off the floor, back off a bit. Practice Baby Cobra, with just a slight lift of the chest, until you feel ready to proceed.

Inhale. Exhale and press back to Downward-Facing Dog or Child's Pose. Hold there for three to five breaths, watching the opening in your back and heart space.

Setu Bandha Sarvangasana: Bridge Pose

Lie on your back with your knees bent, feet on the floor hip-width distance apart, and your arms resting comfortably beside your hips. Breathe and feel the support beneath you. Let your spine be neutral, neither pressing flat to the mat nor overarching.

Bend your elbows and point your hands to the sky, palms in, like robot arms. Breathe. Gently press the back of your head and upper arms into the floor as you lift your chest and roll your shoulders under your back. Stay here for a breath or two, feeling into the engagement in your upper back and opening in your chest. Lift your chin away from your chest to soften your throat and open your breathing.

This is a beautiful way to begin your practice of Bridge Pose. If you wish to proceed further, press your feet down and lift your hips. At this point, the only parts of your body touching the mat should be your feet, backs of upper arms, and head. Your spine is completely lifted off the floor.

As you breathe, extend from the roof of your mouth up through your heart, out through your legs, and down into your feet. If you feel compression in your lower back, gently hug your knees to engage your inner thighs and release the excessive bracing in your gluteal muscles.

As the muscles engage, the body is challenged. As you breathe, welcome into your awareness someone you love or perhaps someone who challenges you. Extend lovingkindness to that person, noticing how it affects your posture.

Stay here for three to five breaths, and then lower down. Pause with your feet on the floor and perhaps bring your knees to touch.

Modification: Supported Bridge Pose

One of my favorite ways to practice this asana is to place a block under the hips so the pelvis is supported. This is an excellent modification to practice in place of or in addition to the pose as outlined above. Here the chest remains lifted, with the shoulder blades drawing in like a pillow to bolster the heart, and the feet firmly on the floor. Allow the arms to rest on the ground with palms face up.

With a block under the sacrum, there is a tangible sensation of being cared for and welcomed just as you are right now. You do not have to be any more or less than you are in this moment. All of you is loved and honored in this place.

Apanasana: Knees-to-Chest Pose

Lower your hips to the floor (if you've practiced Bridge Pose with a block, move it out of the way). Inhale and draw your knees in toward your chest. Wrap your hands or arms around your shins to give yourself a loving hug. Rock side to side or just stay still, breathing here for as long as you'd like.

When you are ready, roll to one side and pause there, breathing deeply. Then press up to a comfortable seat. Place your hands on top of your heart and breathe into this space, giving loving hospitality to whatever resides here at this moment.

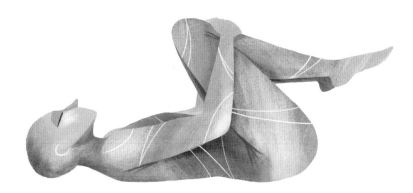

6 Daily Rhythms
Balance in Ordinary Routines

For we need to remind ourselves of this very basic
and very modest fact that we are essentially rhythmic
creatures, and that life needs this rhythm and balance if it is
to be consistently good and not drain from us the precious
possibility of being or becoming our whole selves.

—Esther de Waal

Every summer my family and I spend one week at Kanuga, an Episcopal retreat center in the Blue Ridge Mountains. It is a time for kinship, rest, and renewal. The kids run wild through the fields, hike among old rhododendrons that curve like archways to a sacred temple, and swim in lake water untouched by chlorine. The fresh mountain air does for our bodies what the lush forests and soft vistas do for our minds. The pace of the day is slow and rhythmic, with the relaxed schedule revolving around communal meals prepared by the center's staff. There are options for structured prayer and worship, nature walks, arts and crafts, games, and family events. A quiet time is observed after lunch. There is a slow rhythm to the day that resets the body, mind, and spirit in accordance with the pace of the earth rather than the frenetic demands of modern life.

As humans living in a post-industrial, global society, we have electric lights that extend daytime hours, clocks that drive our comings and goings, and devices that monitor how many steps we've taken in a day and give us up-to-the-second status reports on our vital signs. We have become so divorced from nature's rhythms that it is easy to see ourselves as set apart from, rather than interwoven with, the rhythms of day and night and the cycle of seasons. But instead of measuring our days against the linear digits on a clock or exercise app, what if we could shift toward a wholistic computation of our sense of vitality in relationship to the rise and fall of the day?

To be clear, I'm not advocating an abandonment of technology or a rejection of the abundant benefits of Western medicine and its calculations. What I am proposing is that we integrate these things with the wisdom of nature, which is written into the traditions of yoga and the Rule.

The Rule was written in the context of an agrarian society. Monks, like many people, made their living from working the land. Time was measured by the rising and setting of the sun, and candle- and firelight provided the only illumination beyond that of the moon and stars. The schedule of the day was set in intentional rhythms of prayer, work, study, and rest. Eight times a day the monks would stop what they were doing and join together in worship and prayer. Hours were set aside for the study of Scripture and other sacred texts so that life centered on Christ, not productivity. Meals were simple, and time for silence and sleep prescribed. Benedict gave his monks the great gift of simplicity rather than austerity.

"They should so regulate and arrange all matters that souls may be saved, and members may go about their activities without justifiable grumbling," Benedict writes in the Rule. In short, we must honor bodily needs so the mind and heart may be free and attentive to the presence of God in all aspects of life.

We would do well to remember this. It may seem impossible, and indeed it requires commitment, but we can regulate and arrange our matters so that our souls and the souls of others are uplifted. We can orchestrate our days in accordance with the wisdom of nature.

Ayurveda: The Science of Life

Ayurveda is the traditional system of wholistic medicine in India, so inter-woven with yoga that the two are often considered sisters. Ayurveda, which means "the science of life," is a five-thousand-year-old way of approaching well-being that focuses on proactively creating health before disease and imbalance sets in. The Ayurvedic sages used their finely tuned skills of pattern recognition to observe the rhythms and qualities of nature as they exist in the world and in our bodies. Several basic concepts of Ayurveda will inform our reorientation toward balance:

- Life exists in rhythms and patterns.
- Each pattern contains specific qualities that tend to exist with one another.
- Like qualities increase like qualities.
- Opposite qualities decrease or balance each other.

These qualities are best understood in three categories of being, called *doshas*. A dosha is an interplay of elements and collection of qualities that tend to exist together. There are three doshas: *vata*, *pitta*, and *kapha*. Ayurveda names five elements as the building blocks of nature: space, earth, fire, water, and air. The three doshas are energies that combine these elements in various ways. Understanding them can help us understand ourselves and our daily rhythms.

Vata is the dosha of space and air. Think for a moment of the qualities of space and air. Outer space is cold and expansive. Air moves. Unless imbued with moisture, air is dry. Without pollution, it is clear. Space and air are subtle, not dense. So the main qualities of vata are: cold, moveable, clear, expansive, dry, and light. This collection of qualities gives vata the energy of motion. Vata is the dosha associated with the mind.

Pitta is the dosha of fire and water. Fire is hot, sharp, spreading, intense, and active. Water is flowing and, when uncontaminated, clear. The main qualities of pitta are: hot, sharp, oily, flowing, intense, and active. Pitta, the energy of transformation, is connected to the spirit.

Kapha is the dosha of earth and water. Earth, when not warmed by the sun, is cool. Earth is dense, steady, heavy. There is a softness to earth, and a serenity. And as we noted, water is flowing, smooth, and wet (this is obvious but noteworthy, as it stands in opposition to the dry quality of air). As a whole, kapha is: cool, wet, cloudy (think earth and water mixing together to make mud), fluid, dense, stable, heavy, smooth, soft, and serene. Kapha is the energy of condensation. It is the dosha associated with the body.

The Doshas at Work in the World

The doshas, like the elements of space, earth, fire, water, and air, exist at all times. They are not tangible things but forces at work in your body and in the world, resulting from the interplay of the five elements. Imbalance happens when one or more of the elements exists in greater or lesser proportion than the others. There is no magic formula or specific numerical value ascribed to each element that equals perfect harmony. The doshas, like balance, are in continual, dynamic conversation. It is the conversation and its setting that is important.

Imagining and naming the energy of a particular time of day can help us find sacred, natural rhythms written into time rather than forcing artificial ones. Many of us do not have the luxury of scheduling our days according to the rhythm outlined below, particularly those who work shifts or multiple jobs; however, it is still possible to study the cyclical patterns of a day and find ways to apply this wisdom to your daily rhythm.

Think through the general timeline of a day. It may help to think of the face of an analogue, or circular clock rather than a digital one. What are the qualities of the various times of day?

> **Early morning to sunrise (2:00 a.m.–6:00 a.m.): *Vata*.** In the first hours of the day, the air is cooler than it will be when the sun rises. There is a subtle charge in the atmosphere. Vata is mind mode, and this is acutely expressed during REM sleep, when the conscious and subconscious are engaged in dreaming. When there's an imbal-ance, we may frequently find ourselves waking up and being overrun by racing thoughts. Because of the subtle, cooler, mind mode nature of these hours, this is the traditional time of day for rising early for prayer, study, and meditation.

> **Sunrise to midmorning (6:00 a.m.–10:00 a.m.): *Kapha*.** There's a lush, gentle, fluid quality to the time during and after sunrise, as the birds sing and mist lingers in the air. The world wakes up with

easy movement, and we are invited to do the same. Morning is the perfect time to exercise, practice asana, and eat a healthy breakfast. Sleeping in too late can invite a kaphic imbalance, which we may experience as sluggishness. Rising at an appropriate hour gives the body a sweet, grounded energy to begin the day. For those who have been awake since vata time, the shift into kapha may be when we are finally able to fall back to sleep for a bit before rising.

Midmorning to midafternoon (10:00 a.m.–2:00 p.m.): *Pitta*.

Midmorning is when things really heat up. The day warms, and the energy of the world is awake. Appointments, meetings, errands, work: everything is active and moving. This is fire time, pitta time. The demands of the day come on fast, and we are taking in a million different bits of sensory data and transforming them into useful information. Digestive fire is strong, so it is a good time to eat denser food and fuel the body and mind for the remaining activities of the day. In Western culture, pitta is the time of day during which we become so wrapped up in activities that fire can bring us out of balance and we may become frantic or so task-oriented that we forget about people and prayer.

Midafternoon to early evening or sunset (2:00 p.m.–6:00 p.m.):

Vata. After the sun reaches its peak, there's a tipping point, when the vata forces of air and space return to the forefront of the world. If we've eaten well and either taken a little rest or a little movement to keep the fire of pitta in check, the mind settles clearly into the remaining tasks at hand. This is a good time for communication, writing, and study. Physical and mental activity are at their peak. It's appropriate to keep the body moving at a sustainable pace, keeping in mind that too much activity can be depleting.

Early evening or sunset to late evening (6:00 p.m.–10:00 p.m.): *Kapha.* Once again the light, airy vata surrenders to the grounding, nurturing qualities of kapha. It is time to release the quick activities of the day and return to a place of rest. When we try to extend the intensity of pitta activities that characterize midday through our afternoon and evening, and when we commit to too many activities, we invite airy vata to fuel pitta's fire, which can lead to burnout. Taking our cue from the doshas as much as possible, we can choose evening activities well. Finding things that bring pleasure and refresh the mind allows the overworked nervous system to calm as we embrace the earthy, kapha energy of the evening and prepare for rest.

Night (10:00 p.m.–2:00 a.m.): *Pitta.* Here is pitta, the energy of transformation seen in the metabolic cleansing and renewal processes at their strongest. Food and experience are digested. Sleeping at this time brings the most rest to the body. We may notice that if we stay up too late it becomes more difficult to fall asleep.

When we align ourselves with this ebb and flow of the energies of the day, we create space to listen to the conversation of the doshas in ourselves. Whether or not we have the choice to align our days according to the rhythm of sunrise and sunset, learning about the natural cycles of the day can help us cultivate practices that support our health and well-being in whatever schedule and season of life we are in. For example, as you observe the quality of your waking energy, perhaps you notice that you tend to be more frenzied and disconnected during pitta times of day. You could then make a commitment, as much as possible, to find ways to pause, breathe, pray, or consciously slow your pace to cultivate a better balance between work and spirit.

Benedict's Order of the Day

While Benedict was likely never exposed to Ayurveda, he was so attuned to the rhythms of nature and of the body that his order for the day mirrors the twenty-four-hour cycle of the doshas. It is important to remember that in Benedict's time, one day was measured from sundown to sunup—approximately 6:00 p.m. to 6:00 a.m.

The monks' schedule revolved around eight times for communal prayer—a practice called the Divine Office, or Liturgy of the Hours. Each activity began with a period of communal prayers that included the psalmody and other scriptural readings.

>**Vigils: Middle of the night. Inner vata, mind mode.** Benedict's Rule instructs the monks to "rise at the 8th hour of the night" so that "the community can arise with their food fully digested," and to gather for prayer, followed by a period of reading and study. This was around 2:00 a.m. Having gone to bed near 6:00 p.m., the monks would have slept for eight hours before rising to capitalize on complete digestion and the vata energy of the day.

>**Lauds: Dawn. Outer kapha, body mode.** After their period of reading and study, the monks began the work of the day. The morning kapha cycle is an ideal time for physical movement, because the body is refreshed and the fire of movement and work keeps at bay the kaphic tendency toward stagnation.

Prime: Early morning. The morning's work is put on pause for a brief liturgy to center the mind and heart in prayer. Prime occurs within the kapha time of day, reminding us to keep the needs of the spirit and the needs of the body in balance.

Terce: Morning, around 10:00 a.m. Early pitta energy of transformation. After work during the kaphic period, the monks returned to reading and study, utilizing the focused energy of a body fueled by movement while not overdoing the work.

Sext: Noon. High pitta. This is when the monks ate the first meal of the day (except during times of fasting). The monks ceased their work or reading and gave their bodies nourishment. By doing so, they capitalized on the digestive fire at this time but held it in balance by returning to reading and rest until about 2:30 p.m.

None: Mid-afternoon. External vata time, mind and body mode in harmony. After a period of rest and nourishment via the midday meal, the monks returned to work for a few hours.

Vespers: Late afternoon and evening. Inner kapha, body mode at rest. Now the monks enjoyed a gentle supper. On fast days this may have been the only meal of the day. Then they began a period of rest.

Compline: Night. Inner kapha moving to inner pitta. After the brief and beautiful service of Compline, the monks entered a period of silence. This released them into a time of inner illumination before retiring to bed after sundown. During sleep, then, their bodies were rejuvenated, and their minds and spirits could experience an internal integration of the work and study of the day.

The specific time for each activity and its corresponding length was adjusted throughout the seasons. This adjustment accommodated for the lengthening and shortening of days, which we will explore in the next chapter.

For most of us, rising at 2:00 a.m. to pray and study, putting in a full day's work, and then retiring by 8:00 p.m. would be impossible. Yet the wisdom of the doshic rhythms and Benedictine call to pause for prayer can still be integrated into our daily lives. This can be done by adopting a simple *dina charya*—a daily rhythm. But first, it is important to make an accurate assessment of the current rhythms of our days. We can use deep listening to locate opportunities for change.

Questions for Reflection

What does a typical day look like? Reflect on the rhythms of a regular day, considering which parts of the daily routine feel good and which ones don't. We may not have control over all parts of our schedules, but sometimes we can make adjustments that provide space for prayer and life-giving practices.

Morning

- What time do I rise?
- With which activities do I begin my day?
- Do my mornings feel rushed or nourishing?
- What do I want to make room for? What could I let go of or adjust to make that space?

Midday

- Do I take time to eat a nourishing lunch?
- Does my lunch leave me feeling hungry and spacey? Sluggish and tired?
- Have I lost a sense of purpose and connectivity I may have had upon rising?

Late Afternoon and Evening

- What time do I set aside work?

- What activities am I committed to in the evening?

- Do my evening commitments feel rushed and draining or life-giving?

- What time do I eat dinner?

- Do I often snack until bedtime?

Night

- What time do I go to bed?

- What activities do I engage in before going to bed?

- Do I take some time to be quiet before bed, or do I continually feed my brain with media, communication, or work?

Wellness Practice: Hone Daily Rhythms

Let's look at some ways to attune ourselves to the natural rhythms of the day. Some practices of this dina charya—daily rhythm—may be easy for you to implement; others may be unrealistic for the current season of your life. Take stock and do what you can. Even adopting one or a few of these practices can enhance your sense of balance. Remember: Easy does it. Progress, not perfection.

The outline on the next page is based on a traditional workday. If you work in shifts that include twelve-hour days or overnight hours, or if you are a caregiver with irregular or constant responsibilities, you may still be able to adapt this practice to your current routine where appropriate, keeping in mind the doshic daily cycles.

Be early to bed, early to rise. As much as possible, rise between 5:00 a.m. and 7:00 a.m. and retire by 10:00 p.m. This will allow for adequate sleep and proper digestion.

Move your body, feed your mind, and nourish your soul. Make some time for movement each day; even a few simple stretches will do. Look out the window to observe the quality of the day. Perhaps read a daily devotional, a bit of poetry, or scripture. Journal. Enjoy a few deep breaths. If possible, meditate for five minutes (or more!).

Stimulate your digestion and lymph. Begin the day by drinking hot water and eating a nourishing breakfast to stimulate your digestion, cleanse your body, and fuel your day. Try to eat enough to keep you full until lunch. If you shower in the morning, you could incorporate oil massage or dry brushing.

Take a midday pause. Take a break for lunch. Pause to pray or give thanks for the food you are about to receive, and try to recall the devotional, poetry, or Scripture you read in the morning. Eat a good amount of food so that you feel energized until mid- or late afternoon. This can also be a good time to take a walk or connect with good friends or colleagues—or, if you're able, to take a nap!

Do a midafternoon refresh. If you are hungry, choose a healthy snack. Pause to stretch, or pray for a loved one.

Be intentional about your evening. Finish work by 6:00 p.m. whenever possible. Choose your evening commitments with care to avoid overexertion. Do something that brings you joy: taking a walk, doing a craft, cooking, meeting friends, watching a little TV, or going to your child's baseball game. Read a book. Eat a simple, light dinner, and close the kitchen when finished. Say a prayer before your meal. Give your body time to digest before going to bed.

Prepare for bedtime. Turn off your screens thirty minutes before going to bed to give your brain time to adjust and prepare for sleep. If you shower at night, incorporate oil massage or dry brushing. Journal or read. Close your eyes and welcome a few deep breaths, giving thanks for the day.

Meditation: Cycle of the Day

This is a simple meditation on the doshas as they cycle through the day. It is meant to draw you into your own intuitive understanding of the rise and fall of energy and light. Imagining a day as it moves from dawn to dusk and back again can help us identify the natural rhythms and place ourselves more fully within them.

Sit comfortably in a chair or on the floor. If possible, sit outside, or open a window to let in the fresh air so that you can connect more deeply with the natural world. Turn your attention to the rise and fall of your breath.

Begin by naming the time of day of this moment. Is it morning, afternoon, evening, or night? What is the quality of the energy during this time? Is it calm, frenetic, warm, cool, soft, hard? Without too much analysis, feel your way into as many descriptive words as possible.

Next, turn your attention to the idea of morning. If you're meditating in the morning, stay here. If it is another time of day, use your imagination and memory to recall the sensations of morning. Awaken as much detail of morning as possible—not so much the activities you do in the morning, but the quality of the day. How does the morning air feel? What is the temperature, the color of the light? Is there moisture in the air? Morning is kapha time. See if you can locate the interplay of earth and water during these hours. Notice the sense of possibility and opening that the new day brings.

Now move your awareness to midmorning through midafternoon. How does the world feel? What is the temperature, the light, the strength of the sun? Does the air feel charged or soft? This is pitta time. Wander through the sights and sounds of the hours of midday to find the elements of fire and water.

Begin to settle into midafternoon to evening. How has the day shifted—the light, the sound, the energy? Is it light or heavy? Does the energy feel grounded or changing? This is vata time, when information and energy are carried to finish out the work of the day. If you could pick a color that describes this time of day, what would it be? How do you notice the element of air moving through the afternoon?

Slide your imagination into evening. Work is done, and the air is cooling. There may be much to do before retiring to bed, but notice the invitation to settling offered during this second round of kapha time. How are you embraced and nurtured after the movement of the mind, body, and spirit during the daylight hours? How do the elements of earth and water show up once again?

What is the feeling of night when your body is at rest? Imagine all the restorative processes occurring in your body as it digests food, distributes nutrients, absorbs sensory input, and moves through dreams. How do the transforming qualities of fire manifest as you sleep?

Now move into early morning. Notice the subtle energy of spaciousness, as though all the elements of your being are carried across the expanse of space.

What do you dream? If this is a time of night when you wake without meaning to, notice the rapid movement of thought, however unpleasant. Vata time is moveable, shifting, and open to the subtle realms of being. What would it feel like to light a candle and pray?

Return to the memory of sunrise. Feel the release of the subtle aspects of vata as they sink to the earth for a new day to begin.

Asana Practice: Sun Salutation

Surya Namaskar, or Sun Salutation, is a classic sequence of asanas often done at the beginning of a formal practice as a warmup, as links between other poses, or as a stand-alone practice. Sometimes it is also referred to as a *vinyasa*. Vinyasa is a generic term for a linked series of poses that flow from one to the next, in coordination with the breath and with little pause in between.

Sun Salutation is a wonderful way to practice moving in a rhythm and getting in touch with your body's optimal pace for that moment. Sun Salutation can be done quickly or slowly. Like all of the practices you have done thus far, moving in partnership with breath is key. Because Sun Salutations are to be repeated multiple times in succession or in between other asanas they are a lovely tool for cultivating a cyclical mindset that resonates with the recurring rhythms of the day.

There are two versions of Sun Salutations: Surya Namaskar A, which does not include any lunge poses, and Surya Namaskar B, which includes Warrior I or a variation. We'll do a modified version of Surya Namaskar B that opts for Crescent Pose, which is a little easier than Warrior I. I've included Plank Pose because it is excellent for building heat and core strength and aids in the transitions from standing to the floor. A modification is offered. However, you may also omit the pose if you prefer.

I'll guide you in greater detail through the sequence below, but the general flow of movement and breath in Surya Namaskar is this:

- Begin with **Mountain Pose**.
- Inhale and extend arms up. Exhale and release to **Standing Forward Fold**.
- Inhale, look forward; exhale, bow in.
- Inhale, then step back to **Plank**. Exhale, lower down to the floor.
- Inhale, press up to **Cobra**.
- Exhale, stretch back to **Downward-Facing Dog**.
- Inhale, step one foot forward, and lift your arms up into **Crescent Lunge**. Exhale and settle.
- Inhale, step back to **Downward-Facing Dog.** Exhale and settle.
- Inhale and step the other foot forward and lift into **Crescent Lunge.** Exhale and settle.
- Inhale, step back to **Downward-Facing Dog.** Exhale and settle here for three to five breaths.
- Inhale, step feet to hands for **Standing Forward Fold.** Exhale and bow in.
- Inhale, rise up to standing. Exhale, stand in **Mountain Pose.**
- Repeat the cycle three to five times.

That is a general rhythm of breath and movement. Your breath pattern may be different with a change in postures, happening more on the exhale than the inhale, or vice versa. You may enjoy several rounds of breath before moving to the next pose, or you may move from pose to pose in rapid succession. Again, what is paramount is how you listen to your body and connect its movements to the rhythm of your breath.

Tadasana: Mountain Pose to Uttanasana: Standing Forward Fold

Begin in Mountain Pose. Stand well with your feet hip-width distance apart and parallel. Relax your arms and shoulders, soften your face, and turn your attention to your body. Feel the beating of your heart and the rhythm of your breath.

With your inhale, sweep your arms overhead as though you are welcoming in the first energy of the day. Exhale and lower them back down to settle into the moment. Repeat this several times with your movement following in the wake of the breath, so that your pace becomes rhythmic and aligned with the cycles of your breath.

On your next inhale, sweep your arms up again and stretch out through your fingers to awaken every part of your body. Then exhale and fold forward into Standing Forward Fold. Inhale, and lift from your hips to look forward. Then exhale and bow in.

Palankasana: Plank Pose

Place your hands on the mat shoulder-width distance apart, with your wrist creases parallel to the front of the mat and your fingers spread wide. Move your feet back, step by step, until you are in a push-up position. Keep your knees lifted, with your hips about as high as your shoulders. For a modified pose, you may lower your knees to the floor for support.

Inhale, shift your weight forward so that your shoulders move above and in front of your fingers, and exhale while you lower your body down so that your stomach is on the floor.

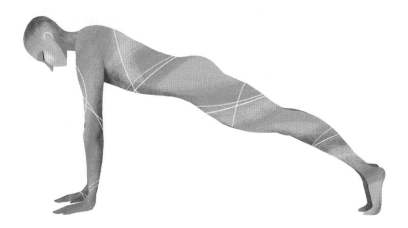

Bhujangasana: Cobra Pose

With your hands on the floor alongside your chest, welcome in a full breath as you soften your belly. Inhale and press the tops of your feet down to root into a strong foundation. Lift your shoulders toward your spine. Exhale and soften through your chest.

Keeping your shoulders back, press your hands down as you inhale and lift your belly and chest off the mat. Exhale. Depending on your comfort level, you may simply lift your chest an inch or so off the mat for Baby Cobra. Do what feels right for your body.

Adho Mukha Svanasana: Downward-Facing Dog Pose

Inhale, tuck your toes, and shift your hips back to your heels to move through Child's Pose before lifting up into Downward-Facing Dog. To begin gently, you may start Downward-Facing Dog with bent knees. Or perhaps "walk it out" by bending one knee and stretching the opposite leg to straight, then repeating. When you are ready, and if it's okay for your lower back, stretch both legs to straight. Firm your arms into the midline to draw in the fullness of your rhythm.

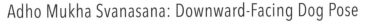

Ashta Chandrasana: Crescent Lunge Pose

Step your right foot forward between your hands to come into a lunge position. You can use one hand to help you step your foot forward.

Make your stance long enough so that your knee is directly over your ankle and your toes are facing forward, with back toes tucked under. Press your feet down into the mat to steady your foundation. Reach your arms forward and lift up into Crescent Lunge Pose. With each inhale, gather the energy of the day to your core. With every exhale, soften and extend out to meet the pulse around you.

With your next exhalation, lower your hands to the mat and step back to Downward-Facing Dog. Inhale, and step the left foot forward to repeat Crescent Lunge Pose on the second side. Exhale when complete and make your way to Downward-Facing Dog.

Stay in Downward-Facing Dog for three to five breaths.

Step your feet forward to your hands for Standing Forward Fold. Root from your pelvis down through your feet as you inhale and rise up to standing. Exhale and release your hands down to the side. Stand in Mountain Pose.

This is one round of Sun Salutations. Repeat this several times, moving slowly or quickly, as your energy dictates. The key here, as in all the poses and sequences, is to move with the rhythm of your breath. Breath begins; movement follows. Listen to the rhythm and allow it to guide you.

Seasonal Rhythms
Balance in the Midst of Change

Spring, summer, autumn, and winter each have particular

gifts and invitations. . . . We recognize the rhythms

of nature as the rhythms of our own soul.

—Christine Valters Paintner

There are many ways to delineate the seasons of the year: school schedules, holidays, the calendar, and the weather. Benedict marked the wheel of the year primarily by the liturgical calendar, moving from Lent through Easter to Pentecost and back again. Interwoven with the yearlong cycles of prayer, fasting, and feasting was a consideration of the cycles of nature.

To accommodate the changing rhythms of the seasons with their variations in temperature, portions of day and night, and types of work to be done, Benedict made adjustments to the daily schedule. In the summer, he allowed the monks to go to bed a little later, shortening the time between vigils and lauds. This allowed the monks to get adequate sleep when the daylight hours lengthened. He also increased the meals to two a day on non-fast days, or when it was especially hot, to provide proper sustenance for work in the fields. In the darker, colder months, the monks went to bed closer to sunset at 6:00 p.m., rising at 2:00 a.m. for vigils, followed by a longer period of readings before lauds at daybreak. There may have been only one meal, but it would have been hearty and earlier than that of the summer supper. "Always let the meal be so scheduled that everything be done by daylight," Benedict wrote. In all seasons, evening was a time for rest and silence.

Seasonal Rhythms of the Body and Soul

Think back to the qualities of space, air, earth, fire, and water that make up the doshas as we explored their alignment with the rise and fall of the day. We can apply this same perspective to our physical, mental, and emotional makeup, as well as to the physical and spiritual invitations of the seasons of the year and the seasons of life. Indeed, this understanding of how we express the doshas in our body, mind, and spirit at any given stage is central to finding balance within Ayurveda's holistic framework. Similar to the way that personality tests can illuminate human nature, doshas can offer a pathway toward understanding ourselves, the seasons of our growth and development, and our relationship to the rhythms of nature.

Each one of us is born with all three doshas, manifesting to greater or lesser degree the building blocks of space, air, earth, fire, and water. How these elements interact with one another informs our tendencies toward balance and imbalance. While we are all born with all three energies, a dominant dosha often emerges in each person. Just as the doshas are associated with different parts of the day and seasons of the year, different doshas are also associated with the many stages of life.

Keep in mind that in regard to the seasons of the year, what follows is based on a North American or European perspective. Climates that have rainy seasons and dry seasons as primary indicators of change still contain the doshas. For example, the rainy season would align with kapha and the dry season with vata or pitta, depending on temperature. Cold and dry tend to be more vata in nature, while hot and dry are more characteristic of pitta. When working with the doshas, it is important to let the way the qualities of space, air, earth, fire, and water are interacting in the environment guide your exploration of nature's rhythms.

Regardless of climate or geography, knowing how the elements and doshas are expressed in your own makeup provides a powerful tool to engage with the seasons of life, the rhythms of the year, and the movement of the spirit.

Spring: Kapha. As winter thaws, water becomes the predominant element mixing with earth to create mud. Rain nurtures budding leaves and flowers. There is a sweet newness in the air as the earth blossoms and brightens after the long, dark days of winter. Internally there is a feeling of awakening and rebirth; a sense that, yes, dreams are possible, and support is available to make them happen.

A person with a predominantly kapha makeup is generally more physically substantial (think muscles and bones, not necessarily weight, though kaphas do gain weight with greater ease than the other types). Kaphas tend to be stable in mood and emotions, nurturing, and reliable. The kapha mind may be slower to absorb information, but once learned, it is learned for life. Because of the element of water, people with a primarily kapha constitution tend to be more easygoing and fluid than the more driven pitta or the more nervous vata. In excess, however, water mixes with earth to become sluggish, and so kaphas also face a stronger potential for inertia.

In terms of seasons of life, kapha is connected to childhood. Kapha tendencies are more pronounced from birth through age twelve, when children are in the building stages of life.

On the level of spirit, kapha is associated with planting seeds and watching them germinate. In the springtime of the soul, we begin to move out of periods that may have been difficult, long, tiring, and frustrating. Just when it may seem that life is at its darkest, a glimmer of light begins to shine. We move into a stage of hope for the future and joy in the present as we start to notice our own rebirth.

Summer: Pitta. With the strength of the summer sun, the predominant element of summer is fire. Days are long, bright, and hot. This a very active time of year for humans, plants, and animals. We take to the water and the woods and the garden, tending to the abundance offered during this time of fruitfulness.

Fiery pitta types tend to be of medium build with bright eyes and big dreams, which they pursue with great intensity. Running hot, they are passionate but also quick to anger. Pittas take in information quickly and have a decent memory, though not one as long-lasting or complete as their kapha friends. They have a love-hate relationship with heat, tending toward intolerance of the summer sun while also enjoying a little spice in their food.

Pitta is a very active dosha and represents age twelve through late middle age: the time of life when we set goals and strike out to make our mark on the world.

During the internal seasons of fire, we are alive with energy. Pitta is a time for passion and action as we work to pursue our dreams. Like the abundant summer harvest, we also see the fruits of our effort. There is a clarity to these periods when the light of our awareness shines bright and we seem to instinctively know what to do and how to respond.

Fall and Winter: Vata. Fall is a transition season that invites us to move from the fire and energy of summer toward a time for gathering in the last fruits of the harvest, followed by rest and release into the dark days of winter. The heat of summer accumulates, leaving a dry quality to the earth manifested in colorful leaves, clear autumn skies, and brisk winds that usher in the cold days to come. Darkness returns, and with it comes the yearning to slow down and turn inward.

Like the weightlessness of space and air, people with a predominantly vata makeup have a lighter build (although not necessarily lighter in weight). A person of a primarily vata constitution has a mind that moves like wind quick in thought, able to connect endless streams of information and retain it well in the short term, although not necessarily far into the future. The expansive quality of space leads to creativity and a greater attunement to the subtle aspects of existence. Vatas tend to be sensitive, which can lead to intuition and insight as well as a marked tendency toward restlessness, fear, and anxiety.

Late middle age to death is the vata time of life, when the body dries out and the fire energy of prior decades turns inward to illuminate deeper layers of experience.

Embracing a vata season of the soul means taking time to rest, contemplate, and, like a field in winter, lie fallow. Vata is both a time of trust in the midst of the unknown and a period of deep reflection and perhaps revelation. Wisdom is found in this liminal space.

In chapter 3 we posed the question, "What season of life am I in, and what does that mean for now, for today?" Just as the seasons move with the calendar year, they also move with our lives. Naming the season in which we find ourselves, on external and internal levels, can help us choose how to use our energy and gifts.

During certain times of life, maybe a few months or years, it can seem that all we are doing is planting seeds and awaiting the harvest. At other times, life is flowing and abundant with the fruits of our effort. Still, other seasons are times of waiting, resting, incubating, and discerning. Forcing the need for fruit during such periods can result in discouragement. Continually moving and pushing and trying to achieve or gain at all costs, without allowing contraction, inner reflection, and silence, is destructive. On the other hand, staying still too long or remaining withdrawn or aloof from the world can be a misuse of our God-given gifts. Allow yourself to claim the current season of your life, recognizing that it is part of a cycle and has much to offer.

Benedict and the Liturgical Order of the Seasons

Just as the Ayurvedic perspective of doshas and the cycles of the day can inform our practice, we can learn from Benedict's adjustments for the rhythms of the year, which created an interior and exterior atmosphere oriented toward balance.

Lent: Vata. Beginning in the last depths of winter, Benedict marked the sacred season of penitence and preparation for the Feast of the Resurrection at Easter with fasting and prayer. Recall that winter is a time of vata, a time for turning inward and attuning oneself to the subtle movements of spirit.

Easter: Kapha. Whether early or late in the calendar year, Easter marks the arrival of spring and the beginning of kapha, when the earth thaws, water flows, and new life emerges. We celebrate resurrection, the rebirth of the spirit, and the promise that death is not the final word. The light of Christ is always there to reorient us toward love.

Pentecost: Pitta. The earth warms and the soul is ignited by the fire of the Holy Spirit. In this season in which we remember the coming of the Holy Spirit, we are tasked with putting love into action, aligning ourselves with the passionate drive seen in pitta.

Prayer continues, as it always does for Benedict. As the earth warms and the days move from Easter through Pentecost and the many days after, from kapha to pitta, a meal may be added to nurture and support the greater physical demands of year. Time is still set aside for study and prayer, though with the increase in daylight there are also more hours for other labor.

Advent, Christmas, and Epiphany: This phase of the liturgical year moves through three seasons of the soul. Advent moves with vata, inviting us to turn in and prepare for kapha and the Feast of the Incarnation at Christmas, followed by pitta's glow at Epiphany, when we see Light in the world.

For Benedict, there were always days of fasting in the midst of all liturgical or earthly seasons. Such days call us to remember that all phases of life and nature deserve pause, reverence, and attention.

Questions for Reflection

- Which dosha(s) do you identify with the most? You may want to use the Resources for Further Study at the back of this book to guide you.
- How do you mark the seasons of the year?
- What would it be like to embrace a seasonal perspective to living?
- Using the doshas as a framework, what soul season do you find yourself in?

Wellness Practice: Find Seasonal Rhythms

Even though we express the doshas in our own unique ways, there are some general guidelines for embracing seasonal rhythms that will serve us well in aligning with the patterns of nature. Living into *ritu charya*—seasonal routines—can lead us toward sacred balance.

Spring: Kapha

- Move! Kapha can get stagnant and bogged down. As the body produces more mucus in its own version of a spring thaw, move to get lymphatic fluid and prana flowing clearly. Walk, add some cardio, or begin or intensify your yoga practice. Any movement will do!

- Start the day with hot water to stimulate balancing warmth. Sip it hot or room temperature throughout the day.

- Do oil massage. If you are strongly kapha with a tendency toward oily skin and excess congestion, however, consider switching to or continuing dry brushing.

- Notice the flowering in the world. Listen to the birds and watch as the colors change from muted to bright.

- For kapha seasons of the soul, take note and delight in the many ways you are being reborn. Look for the first signs of germination and blossoming of seeds you may have sown long ago.

Summer: Pitta

- Rest and play. Take time to embrace the energetic fire of this season. Play outdoors, or use the intensity to work on a project or increase your physical strength. Be sure to balance all the extra effort with plenty of rest. Sit in the shade, or rest on or near a body of water.

- Start the day with hot water. Sip it room temperature (or hot, if you prefer) throughout the day. Ice water can be a shock to the body, but if you are outdoors and very hot, give it a try.

- Continue oil massage. If you used a heavy oil such as almond or sesame for oil massage during the winter and early spring months, consider switching to a lighter coconut oil, which is more cooling.

- For pitta seasons of life, enjoy drawing on the extra fire and drive to pursue your dreams. Take care to balance this activity with plenty of rest to avoid burnout.

Fall and Winter: Vata

- Turn inward. As the days grow shorter, now is an excellent time to practice turning inward. Move throughout the day to keep your body active with just enough heat to pacify vata's cold nature. Avoid overexertion, particularly in the evening, so you can savor the grounding, cozy quality of a dark evening.

- Start the day with hot water and sip it throughout.

- Make oil massage a priority. You may continue with coconut oil for as long as feels appropriate (even into the winter months, particularly if you have pitta tendencies), or you could switch to almond or sesame oil. True shea butter, without a lot of additives and unreadable ingredients, is also good for this time.

- Like the gift of good sleep and dreams, there are gifts in the darkness and vata seasons of the soul. Being in a space of unknown can be a profound challenge and also a potent encounter with possibility and wisdom. Allow yourself to explore all that exists in the subtle, the mysterious, the dark, and the difficult, knowing that it may have the power to lead you to new life.

Meditation: Wheel of the Year

This meditation is similar to the one offered in the previous chapter on daily rhythms. The intent is to awaken to the gifts and invitations offered during each season of the year.

Sit comfortably and close your eyes. Keep a soft focus on your breath for a few moments as you settle in. Set an intention to be present to each season of the year, and open yourself to the wisdom each season has to offer.

Begin in spring. Become aware of the buds and blossoms, the bright green of the small, new leaves. Imagine the thaw of frozen rivers and lakes. As the days lengthen, notice the invitation to newness and awakening. Spring brings rebirth. What is being birthed in you? What possibilities are beginning to bloom?

Follow this blooming into summer. The sun is strong and the days are long. Feel the heat and fullness and notice the abundance showing up at farm stands, in gardens, and in your own life. What blossoms are bearing fruit? What fullness, energy, and inspiration do you feel? At the same time, notice if there is an invitation to rest and recreate that accompanies summer's heat. Is there an invitation to wander in the world and marvel at its brilliance?

As summer's heat builds, watch for a period of complete ripening. By mid-summer the days begin to shorten, but the invitation to fullness and play continues. This is when the harvest begins, as you gather in the fruits of summer.

Gradually the heat begins to wane, and a crispness infuses the air. The sky grows clear and bright and leaves change color, igniting the world with the red, orange, and gold of fire. Feel the drying out as winds blow in and sap draws into the center of trees. Fall is a time to gather in and release. Welcome in the harvest of your energy. As the days darken and the leaves fall, turn inward to embrace the dark. Release.

Winter arrives and brings with it darkness and cold. Warm yourself by the fire. Wrap yourself in blankets and accept the invitation to lie fallow and rest in a space of not knowing. Much of the earth is dormant. Yet in this dormancy there is an integration of all that was drawn in. Use the gift of darkness to open to possibility.

Continue to breathe as you watch the cycle of seasons revolve around you. In which season do you feel most comfortable? What season's invitation do you long to accept?

Allow yourself some time to delight in the gifts offered by the elements as they dance through the year. When you are ready, breathe and open your eyes.

Asana Practice: Twisting Postures

The change of seasons—particularly the shift from winter to spring and summer to fall—are periods of intense activity. From winter to spring, that activity is one of budding and building. In contrast, the turn from summer to fall is one of gathering and release. Such profound shifts in energy invite us to change how we interact with the world. We may feel a sudden urge to clear out the closets or get rid of the detritus that has built up over the preceding months. This impulse to clear and create space for what comes next is a natural response to the conversation that happens between the doshas as they move through the wheel of the year.

The weeks in which winter turns to spring and summer turns to fall are excellent for detoxification. Twisting postures aid in detoxification, as they encourage greater blood and pranic flow to the organs. Much like wringing out a dish towel, they "wring out" toxicity in the body. They are also a tonic for the nervous system, energizing us when we feel low and calming us down when we feel agitated.

To twist safely, we must first cultivate steadiness by drawing into the core and the midline. It is around that steady midline that we revolve. It is there that we learn of the ever-present Grace that holds us in the midst of change.

Sukhasana: Easy Pose

As you sit, bring your legs to a gentle, cross-legged position. If your knees are higher than your navel and you feel rounding or tightness in your hamstrings and lower back, elevate your hips by sitting on a block or a few folded blankets. Alternatively, you may sit with your knees bent and your feet on the floor.

Rest your hands comfortably on your thighs and breathe. Sense a vertical axis of steadiness from the crown of your head through your spine and into your pelvis. This is called the *sushumna nadi*, or "channel of the most gracious."

Inhale and draw your attention and muscular energy from all sides of your body into this steady center. Exhale and extend from the center back out.

Apanasana: Knees-to-Chest Pose

Lie on your back and hug your knees in toward your chest. Breathe and roll or rock from side to side, giving a little massage to your spine.

Jathara Parivartanasana: Revolved Abdomen Pose

Stretch your arms out to the side, or bend your elbows into a cactus shape if you prefer. Lower your feet to the floor and gently shift your hips a little to the left. Inhale and collect your energy to the steady Presence in your core, draw your knees in toward your chest, then lower your knees to the right. If you would like additional support, you may place a block or blankets between your knees to help ease tension. Keep both shoulders on the floor. If your opposite shoulder lifts off the floor, back out of the pose and elevate your knees on a block, a pillow, or stack of blankets.

As you breathe, consciously relax around your navel. Soften through the underside of your ribs, allowing constriction in the belly to let go even while it is engaged in the twist.

Stay here for five to seven breaths. Inhale and bring your knees back to your chest, then lower your feet to the floor. It is important to inhale before moving so that you engage gentle muscle energy before releasing the healthy constriction that occurs in a twist.

Shift your hips a couple of inches to the right, draw your knees back in toward your chest, and then lower them to the left, thus repeating the pose on the second side. Inhale to come out of the pose. Pause, then come up to a seated position.

Parivrtta Sukhasana: Seated Twist Pose

Sit on the floor with your legs crossed. If your knees are higher than your navel and you feel rounding or tightness in your hamstrings and lower back, elevate your hips by sitting on a block or a few folded blankets. This is essential, as it will encourage a neutral spine, allowing you to sit up straight and release bracing in the hips.

Inhale and stretch your arms up to the sky. Gently hug in to your midline, then exhale and lower your left hand toward your right knee, placing your right hand behind you. If bringing your left hand to your right knee is too much for your shoulder or your belly, back off and let your hand come to a place of comfort, perhaps on your inner thigh or ankle. Keep the twist small and gentle to avoid over-rotating, which may create tension in the neck and shoulders.

Breathe into your lungs and feel the back of your ribs expand. Relax your shoulders. Stay in the twist for five to seven breaths. Then inhale and lift your arms, returning to the center. Exhale and twist to repeat the pose in the second direction.

Dandasana: Staff Pose

Sitting on your mat, block, or blanket, stretch your legs straight out in front of you. Rotate your legs inward so that the four corners of your knees and your toes face the sky. Press your heels into the mat. Gather strength and stability from your feet up the bones of your legs and into the core of your pelvis, and then exhale from your pelvis and release down. Let your hands rest by your sides, pressing your palms or fingertips into the earth. Find steadiness within the cycles around you.

Parivrtta Marichyasana: Revolved Sage Pose

Remain seated (and elevated, if necessary). Bend your right knee and place your foot on the floor. Depending on your mobility, your foot may be next to your left calf, knee, or inner thigh.

Inhale and lovingly hold your right shin with your left hand as you sit tall. Again, draw in to your midline to stay steady, then exhale and twist to the right. Lower your right hand to the floor or a block behind you. You may keep your left hand or arm wrapped around your knee. Alternatively, you could inhale, stretch up to create space in your belly, and then hook your elbow on the outside of your knee. Be gentle.

Exhale and settle in for five to seven breaths. Soften your gaze. Note the physical season of the world around you—winter, spring, summer, fall. What qualities do you sense outside and within yourself?

Inhale to unwind. Exhale. Pause and repeat on the second side.

Return to Staff Pose, and press into the support of the earth.

Sukhasana: Easy Pose

Bring your legs back to a gentle, cross-legged position and sit quietly for a few breaths. Give thanks for the steadiness that holds you as you embrace the change of seasons in nature, your body, and your life.

8

Silence
Quieting the Footsteps

Silence [is] the source of all being . . .

Silence is the sea that we swim in.

—Barbara A. Holmes

For my first year or two of teaching yoga, I did not play music in class. I found it distracting. After some time, however—and I don't remember why—I began to incorporate instrumental music that mirrored the arc of the sequence. A few years later, I added music with lyrics (only after I was certain I wouldn't want to sing along more than teach). Now music is a routine element in my class.

Yet on occasion, such as when I can't get the stereo to work, I teach without music. After those classes, students give feedback that they didn't miss the music at all. They say things like, "It was just nice to have some more quiet," and, "The silence was refreshing."

In a world full of noise, silence and quiet have become precious commodities. Without periods of intentional silence to keep us in balance, the sounds of the external world and the chatter of our own minds can pull us off center. As an endless stream of loud and invasive stimuli assault our brain, our nervous system kicks into high gear and we have no time to absorb the totality of our days. Without periods of silence, we cannot till the inner environment necessary to listen and respond to God's invitation.

Cultivating silence is like steeping tea. Leaves are placed in the welcoming warmth of water, which draws out their essential flavor, nutrients, and healing properties. What was once dried is transformed. A soft communication happens, and in that communication something new is born.

Taking time to be quiet helps us withdraw to an interior peace, in which we are neither speaking nor listening. We just *are.* Right there in the moment. We become like tea leaves, received by the warmth of Grace and ready to be transformed. Silence for us is a period of resting in Presence and allowing wisdom to seep in.

In his Rule, Benedict instructs that "monastics should diligently cultivate silence at all times, but especially at night." They are to keep silent as much as possible during the day to better concentrate on the work at hand, be it manual labor, prayer, or study, and thus be mindful of the Divine in every moment of life. On top of this, Benedict adds an additional requirement for silence to be kept in the evening. After a period of communal reading and prayer, the monks are to retire in silence, sent to bed on a note of holy inspiration and quiet. The silence is only to be broken with utmost care if the prioress or abbot needs to give an instruction or if a guest needs attention.

Silence is a habit we learn to cultivate. Through practice we learn to shut off the television, close the book, cease our speech, and stop texting. We don't create an absence of noise so much as we reduce the quantity of distraction.

Silence also helps us become better listeners to those with whom we are in relationship. Pausing to be silent while others are speaking gives us the chance to step beyond ourselves and be more present and responsive to our loved ones. We may also find that there is a particular person or group of people we can just be quiet with. Sometimes there is no need for speech. Sometimes we can just exist alongside each other, feeling the fullness of creation in shared presence.

Perhaps the biggest challenge to silence is the fear of what we may find when we get quiet. The anxiety we have kept at bay through busyness shows up in a rapid heartbeat. To-do lists may race through an unquiet mind, as might memories we don't want to relive and fears for the future we thought we had escaped. All these insecurities show up when we first enter into silence.

In silence we meet the parts of ourselves that most need love and hospitality. In silence we have the opportunity to give ourselves the compassion we so desperately seek. And in this compassionate allowance for all parts of ourselves, fear and anxiety start to lose their hold on our sense of self. As we let go, we sink into the great gift of love and listen with what Benedict calls the "ear of the heart."

The physical movements of asana keep the body vital and healthy, so it is not a distraction from the interior work of the mind and soul. The breathwork of pranayama brings the sympathetic (flight or fight response) and parasympathetic (rest and digest response) nervous systems into harmony, which softens and slows a barrage of thought. In doing so, we train ourselves to be mindful of what we are doing. In those moments, non-essential stimuli fall away and we may feel like we are "in the flow." Absorbed in our task, we can savor the moment.

Pratyahara: Tools for Silence in the Modern World

Asana and pranayama are two key functions of yoga. Another function is *pratyahara*, or sensory withdrawal, which is the practice of turning our attention inward. In *The Tree of Yoga*, B. K. S. Iyengar writes that pratyahara is like the bark of a tree, which carries input from the sensory organs of limbs and leaves on its journey to the core. Our senses, when put to good use, are a valuable tool for cultivating silence.

We may create silence by reducing the noise in the physical environment—turning off the TV, closing the door, ceasing our speech. Conversely, we can also create silence by listening to hear—really *hear*—the sounds around us. To see the colors of the room. To taste the flavor of our food.

The tools below are suggestions for pratyahara as a path to rejuvenating, holy silence. Some of these tools may seem more attractive to you or work better than others. Play around with them. Try one and see what happens.

I recognize some of these practices may be more difficult for extroverts than for introverts, who tend to crave silence. Try them anyway. Silence is crucial for balance.

Reduce media

If you listen to the radio or music in the car, turn it off for a trip or two. If you immediately turn on the TV, radio, or a podcast when you get up in the morning or return home at night, try leaving them off. Listen to the sounds in and around your home instead.

Take a reading sabbatical

In *The Artist's Way*, a classic book on reclaiming creativity, Julia Cameron prescribes a week of reading deprivation as a tool for emptying life of distraction and filling the creative well. Given that reading and study are a foundation of Benedictine life, this directive may sound strange. And you will likely not be able to get through an entire day without reading something. Life is full of words! Complete and total deprivation is not the goal here. But try to identify those moments in which you tend to feed yourself with words to avoid just being quiet. Do you always read the news at breakfast instead of savoring the flavors of your food? Do you reach for a novel when you are upset? Do you constantly check your email? I know I often do. See if you can abstain from those practices for a little while. Or if not, delay them. When the urge to escape into fiction strikes, pause, take a few deep breaths, and listen to your thoughts. What arises? If you typically read before bed, try putting the book aside for one week. Instead of reading and filling your brain with more information, shut the light off and just be. Lie in bed and breathe. See how this may calm your evening.

Take a social media fast

Unless social media is part of your job, try committing to a week of freedom from it. Avoid Facebook and Instagram. If you must engage with social media, try to do so only at designated times—and not at bedtime—rather than randomly and frequently throughout the day.

Have a quiet day

If you have the luxury to take a day or half a day at home by yourself, make it a silent retreat. Put the phone on silent and speak to no one. This includes texting. You don't have to abstain from reading or writing or doing laundry if you don't want to. Go about whatever activities you like, but do them in a spirit of quietude. Watch what it feels like not to hear the sound of your own voice.

Attend a centering prayer or meditation group

Silence can also be found in community. Try attending a session or two of a centering prayer or meditation group. Notice the gentle power of sitting in a room with others while neither speaking nor listening.

Questions for Reflection

- What is your relationship to silence? Does it scare you? Do you crave it?
- What is your first response to moments of silence, be they at home, in church, a yoga studio, a conversation?
- Where and when can you create intentional moments of quiet in your day? Remember that silence is not the total absence of noise.
- What sounds help you move to a space of inner quietude?

Wellness Practice: Practice Four Phases of the Breath

If asana is the gateway to stilling the body, pranayama is the gateway to stilling the mind. When we first get quiet, either to sit for formal meditation or just to reduce distracting noise, it is always helpful to take a few deep breaths. Attentive breathing softens the mind and gives room to be in Presence.

Practicing this Four Phases of the Breath pranayama is an excellent way to draw inward, or practice pratyahara, which leads to deeper absorption. The four phases of pratyahara are:

- **Puraka:** Filling up. Inhalation.
- **Antara Kumbhaka:** The expansive pause after inhalation when the lungs are full with life-giving air. This is a powerful time to open to Presence and silence, as the breath no longer makes a sound.
- **Rechaka:** Releasing. Exhalation.
- **Bahya Kumbhaka:** The suspension when breath is fully emptied before another one begins. This is a time for resting in possibility, waiting to receive God's call.

Technique

- Sit comfortably or lie down. Close your eyes and welcome in a few deep breaths. Slowly begin to turn your attention more fully to your breathing.
- Inhale and hear the sound of air drawing up through your nostrils and filling your lungs.
- Pause.
- Retain the breath for a few counts and notice how your interior expands ever so gently, like a balloon, before releasing into a complete exhalation.
- Pause.
- Watch and wait for your breath to arise again. Listen to what you hear in this space of possibility.

Repeat this pattern for a few rounds, retaining the breath with a bit of intention. Then when you are ready, return to a natural, gentle rhythm of breathing. Observe, listen to, and feel how these four phases, especially the expansive pauses, exist in your breath cycle. Watch as this leads your senses into a place of quiet.

Meditation: Listening to Noise

This is one of my favorite meditations for quieting a barrage of thoughts and external stimuli. It also helps reduce the need to control an environment in order to find silence. The idea is to listen—really listen—to the sounds around you, especially those that seem distracting. Watch as this attentiveness slowly melts distraction into focus and silence and receptivity to wisdom. This can be done in formal meditation, as outlined below, or anywhere and anytime you need a quiet moment.

This meditation is best done upright to avoid falling asleep.

Take a comfortable seat. Close your eyes and feel a few rounds of breath. Turn your attention to the sounds in the room. Listen to the hum of the electronics, the sounds of people around you. Seek out the most distant sound you can hear. Listen as new sounds enter your field of awareness. The air conditioning begins a new cycle. A car passes by. The phone rings. Without resisting or judging any one sound, welcome all this noise into your awareness.

Now start to move your attention to the closest sounds you can hear. The quiet rise and fall of your breath. The gurgling in your stomach. Continue to let your attention soften.

Sit like this for five or ten minutes. You might notice the point at which the noise falls away and you are simply resting in the dynamic silence and space of your heart.

Asana: Yin Yoga

Yin Yoga is an approach that involves long holds that facilitate health and rejuvenation, particularly in the ligaments and bones. *Yin* is a term from the Taoist tradition that refers to cool, interior, and earthy qualities of existence. Yin stands as a complement to the *yang*, which represents the warmer, exterior, and closer-to-the-sky qualities of existence. They mirror the yogic term *hatha*, with *ha* meaning warm and sun-like, and *tha* meaning cool or moon-like. Sun and moon, yin and yang, stability and movement, listening and silence, the dance of opposites: these are the nature of being, and the conversation between them is where we find sacred balance.

The following yin practice is an invitation to slow down and rest in silence as you breathe. Remembering that silence is not the absence of noise, you may notice that as you settle into a yin posture you become more aware of your thoughts or the feelings in your body. That is okay! Silence is a time to absorb and integrate. Consider your yin practice like a cup of tea. By holding a pose and not rushing to what comes next, you allow yourself to steep in Divine quiet, allowing Presence to unfold from within.

You have already become acquainted with the postures in this series throughout the previous chapters. The difference now is that you will be staying in each asana for three to five or even seven minutes. Start small, beginning with three minutes. If you find you can stay longer, do so. If not, shorten the hold to two minutes.

Because you will be holding the posture for some time, back off on your effort by making your shape a little smaller—for instance, not folding as far in a forward fold. When working the poses in a more yang fashion, it is at times appropriate to go to your edge. In yin, however, I invite you to back away from the edge so that the intensity of the pose comes not from the form but from the depth of the internal transformation.

The nature of yin postures can prompt physical, mental, or emotional discomfort. I encourage you to use all the tools and principles you have practiced thus far. Listening can help you discern if there is true pain or mere discomfort. If there is pain, please adjust or move out of the pose. Hospitality can help you welcome your experience, and stability enables you stick with it as you grow in subtle ways. The longer you stay in quiet witness to the dynamics of the posture, the more you may notice a cyclical or rhythmic pattern of bracing and release that occurs without any conscious prompting. This is the power of the pose working through you.

Above all, easy does it. Silence is an act of returning to humility and the Ground of Being.

Balasana: Child's Pose

Begin in Child's Pose. Bring your knees slightly wider than hip-width distance apart. Sit your hips back on your heels. If they cannot comfortably rest there, you may place a blanket under your seat between your hips and your heels. Bow forward and stretch your arms out in front of you, or rest them alongside your hips.

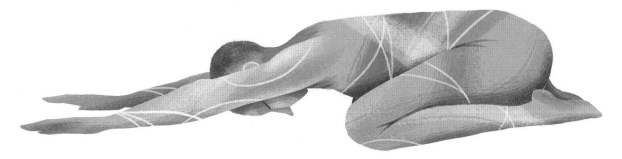

Breathe here for three to five minutes, then slowly come to a seated position.

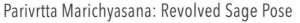

Parivrtta Marichyasana: Revolved Sage Pose

From a seated position (elevated, if necessary, to maintain a healthy inner curve and lift in your lower back), stretch both legs out to straight. Bend your right knee and place your foot on the floor. Depending on your mobility, your foot may be next to your left calf, knee, or inner thigh.

Inhale and hold your right shin with your left hand as you sit tall. Lightly draw in to your midline to stay steady, then exhale and twist to the right. Lower your right hand to the floor or a block behind you.

You may keep your left hand resting on or your left arm wrapped around your knee. Be gentle.

Exhale and settle in for three minutes. Inhale to unwind. Exhale. Pause and repeat on the second side.

Parivrtta Janu Sirsasana A: Extended Head-to-Knee Pose with Side Bend

Extend your legs out in front of you. Inhale, then, keeping your right leg straight, bend your left knee out to the side and bring your left foot in toward your groin. Your knee will be at about a forty-five-degree angle

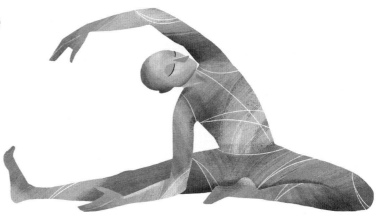

from your hip—or less, if need be. Flex your right foot and rotate the extended leg in so the knee and toes face the sky. Exhale and settle down through your sitting bones.

Place your right arm on your right thigh, the floor, or a block, and stretch your left arm up to the sky. As you raise your left arm alongside your ear, rotate your arm in so the palm faces down. If this causes discomfort, you may bring your left hand to the back of your head and allow your upper arm to rest against the side of your head. Gently press your head into your left hand as though leaning into a soft pillow. This will open your throat and prevent undue strain on your neck. You may also place your left hand on your hip or lower back, palm facing up.

Stay here for three to five minutes, and then repeat on the second side.

Paschimottanasana: East–West Stretch or Seated Forward Fold Pose

From the previous pose, bring your legs back to straight. Check that your knees and toes face the sky. Inhale, flex your feet, and reach your arms up to the sky. Exhale, fold from your hips, and bring your hands to your thighs or to the floor beside your hips, shins, or feet. Only go as far as you can while still breathing with ease.

Allow your attention to be soft as you breathe. Be here for three to seven minutes. When you are ready, inhale and lift back up.

Sucirandhrasana: Eye of the Needle Pose

Lie on your back with your pelvis neutral. Breathe, lift your right foot, and cross your ankle over your left thigh. You may stay like this, or you could place your right hand gently on your right thigh. Breathe and feel the soft sensation in your outer hips and belly. This may be plenty.

If you feel you have the mobility to move further, lift your left foot off the floor and draw your knees in toward your chest. Thread your right hand between your legs and hold the back of your left thigh with both hands. Relax your shoulders.

Breathe here for three to five minutes. Lower both feet to the floor. Pause, then repeat on the second side.

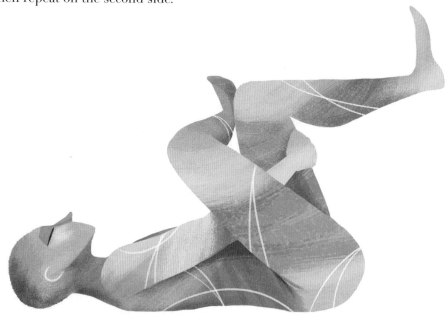

Supported Setu Bandha Sarvangasana: Supported Bridge Pose

Lie on your back with your knees bent, feet on the floor hip-width distance apart, and your arms resting comfortably beside your hips. Breathe and feel the support beneath you. Let your spine be neutral, neither pressing it flat to the mat nor overarching.

Lift your hips and place a block under your sacrum. Bend your elbows and point your hands to the sky, palms in, like robot arms. Breathe. Gently press the back of your head and upper arms into the floor as you lift your chest and roll your shoulders under your back. Lift your chin away from your chest to soften your throat and open your breathing. Lower your arms down and let them rest on the earth, palms face up.

Stay here for three to five minutes, then lower down. Pause with your feet on the floor and perhaps bring your knees to touch.

Jathara Parivartanasana: Revolved Abdomen Pose

Stretch your arms out to the side, or bend your elbows into a cactus shape, if you prefer.
Shift your hips a few inches to the left. Inhale and bring your knees in to your chest. Pause here, then lower your knees to the right. If you would like additional support, you may place a block or blanket between your knees to help ease tension. Keep both shoulders on the floor. If your opposite shoulder lifts off the floor, back out of the pose and elevate your knees on a block, a pillow, or stack of blankets.

Stay here for three minutes. Inhale, bring your knees back to your center, and place your feet on the floor. Shift your hips a couple of inches to the right, then draw your knees in to your chest. Now lower your knees to the left to repeat the pose on the second side.

Savasana: Corpse Pose

Corpse Pose is said to be the most profound and perhaps most difficult yoga posture, because it is one of total surrender. In Corpse Pose there is nothing but stillness and quiet, as the body integrates all the shifts in prana, work of the muscles and bones, and fluctuations of the mind. It reminds us that our time on this earth is finite and that we will one day die. In practicing Corpse Pose, we give up our striving, our effort, our control, and simply rest in infinite Presence.

Remain supine and stretch your arms and legs out long. Let your feet relax out to the side. Gently lift your chest and roll your shoulders under so your shoulder blades are broad and your front body expansive. Turn your arms up. Close your eyes. Breathe and rest here for five to seven minutes.

When you are ready, welcome small movements back to your body, then roll to one side. Pause for a breath or two and then press up to a comfortable seat. Bring your hands together in front of your heart and offer thanks for this time of quiet.

156

Sabbath

Rest along the Way

There is a pervasive form of contemporary violence to which

the idealist most easily succumbs: activism and overwork. . . .

To allow oneself to be carried away by a multitude of conflicting

concerns, to surrender to too many demands, to commit

oneself to too many projects, to want to help everyone

in everything, is to succumb to violence.

—Thomas Merton

In January 2007, I collapsed at work. The illness I had been struggling with since college reached a breaking point. My body was wracked with chronic pain and debilitating fatigue. I was dizzy and depressed, and I couldn't function for more than three or four hours without needing to lie down. I couldn't walk a mile without becoming breathless and drained. Under the care and direction of my doctors I took a medical leave of absence and ultimately never returned to that job.

During this time, I came across the wise words of Thomas Merton quoted on the previous page, and I posted them near my desk at home. They guided my healing journey in the ensuing years and remain an essential compass for me today.

There are seasons of life when work—paid or unpaid, manual or at a desk—demands more hours of the day than we care to give. Attending meetings, childrearing, volunteering, cleaning, caring for sick family members or friends: the activities that require our attention can layer and conflict until we are consumed and exhausted. Not every season can be one of simplicity and spaciousness. But every season, even the most hard-driving, can be one of sacred balance. The trick is knowing how to respond to the particular call of the current season of life.

The principles and practices we've explored thus far are the guideposts for balanced living. Still, there is one more practice essential to sacred equilibrium: keeping the sabbath.

Sabbath comes from the Hebrew *shabbat*, meaning "to cease." It is rooted in the Judeo-Christian idea that on the seventh day God rested. When we practice sabbath alone or with our family, friends, or community, we cease the work of *doing* and make space for rest and renewal in the act of *being*. We are both human beings and human doings. Doing is necessary. Being is necessary to cease the habitual violence of overdoing. The beauty is that you get to decide what *doing* and *being* mean to you.

In *The Rule of St. Benedict: A Spirituality for the 21ˢᵗ Century*, Sr. Joan Chittister writes that we practice sabbath "so that the mundane and the immediate do not become the level of our existence." Sabbath rest from work is a time to reconnect with and reanchor ourselves in the Ground of Being. It is an act of humility that demonstrates our understanding that we are not in charge of the world, that our daily tasks do not define our identity, and that we are created for more than just productivity. As John Valters Paintner writes, "We were also created to be in relationship with our Creator. And that takes time."

In Benedict's day, Sundays were free from manual labor. Parts of the Divine Office were expanded and more time given to study and rest. The sabbath was an intentional time for the community to renew the commitment to Christ by placing even greater emphasis on the heart and soul.

The Benedictine way of balancing work and rest is rooted in a redefinition of work. The primary work is not manual labor; the primary work is the Divine Office and lectio divina. The primary work is the undertaking of putting on the mind of Christ and writing it into the fabric of the heart. Manual labor is recognized as necessary for cultivating a life free from reliance on patrimony, and it is given due reverence. Yet taking a full day off from manual labor is an exercise in stepping beyond the seductive nature of labor as definition of self and sustenance. Keeping the sabbath moves us in a deeper confidence in the provision of God to fulfill the work of the soul.

One of the most insidious terms in business and management circles of today is *work-life balance*. The idea treats the two as if they are separate entities. Work in the office, the factory, the university, the nonprofit, the home fills a significant quantity of the hours of our day. Why, then, is work not considered *part* of life?

I understand the origin of the term. It is an attempt to frame a sense of balance and uphold boundaries between the demands of employment and our lives with family, friends, hobbies, passions, and even religion and spirituality. Perhaps a healthier way of categorizing the hours of the day, however, would be to focus on an interior orientation to what is life-giving rather than life-draining.

Jobs we don't like, toxic family relationships or work environments, a mechanical rush from one task to another: these are triggers that can take us down an enervating path of disconnection from self and Spirit. Sometimes we have to work jobs that aren't our favorite in order to pay for the basic necessities. Sometimes we must engage in relationship with a difficult family member, or fill the calendar with commitments, because that is the call of the moment. But there are boundaries we can set that encourage self-care in the midst of trying times. The practice of sabbath is one.

The ancient tradition of sabbath as a full day off from any work—either on Saturday or Sunday—is virtually nonexistent in our current culture. But that doesn't mean we can't practice sabbath in a manner suitable to our lives as they are. Setting aside time for rest—for an evening, a half day, or a full day—is crucial to our sacred balance. Any small, intentional movement away from the layers of immediate doing can be a form of sabbath. A contemplative walk can become a sabbath. An asana practice can be a sabbath. A moment of pause between activities—statio, which we looked at in chapter 4—can be a mini-sabbath. The essence of sabbath is the reorientation toward the sacred and meaningful in life.

Sabbath as Nonviolence

The first moral tenet, or *yama*, outlined in the Yoga Sutras is *ahimsa*. Ahimsa means nonviolence, non-harming, or the unwillingness to do harm. In ahimsa, we are called to discern what a life of nonviolence means to us and then live in accordance with those values. From ecology to diet to our relationship to social justice, the many layers of depth to ahimsa are deeply personal and transform the way we interact with the world around us. In the context of sabbath, we turn ahimsa inward as the commitment to do no harm to ourselves and embrace a life of love and peace in recognition that we all need rest.

We need time to lie fallow, to mend, to decompress, to recreate, and to nourish our physical and spiritual selves. Even the practices we know are life-giving—our prayer, our exercise, our asana, our good work—can all become part of a draining, rote to-do list. To keep ourselves fresh and clear, we need time to cease. Whether or not our sabbath includes these activities, we need time to reconnect with the practices that keep us in sacred balance.

Delight is a spiritual practice. It is the very thing God does after the creation of the world. Tantric yoga philosophy illuminates the concepts of *ananda* and *lila*. Ananda means Divine bliss—the essential joy of the Creator taking delight in creation and in the lila, or the unfolding play of life. In our intentional moments or hours of sabbath, we savor the delights of life: the fruit of work, the warmth of family and friends, the enjoyment of creative projects, the wonders of nature, a good book, a cuddle—and yes, if at times it serves our need to cease work, a bit of television.

In their course "Monk in the World" at AbbeyoftheArts.com, Christine and John Valters Paintner posit that the delight of sabbath is a sacred, loving, nonviolent act of humility and justice. As slaves in Egypt, the Hebrew people were not allowed to rest. The commandment "Remember the sabbath day, and keep it holy" (Exod 20:8 NRSV) is a life-affirming resistance to oppressive systems that cut us off—intentionally or unintentionally—from the wisdom and beauty of being.

In this life-giving, nonviolent gift of sabbath, we renew not just our commitment to self-care but our ability to love and care for others. I am much more likely to be short-tempered with my young child when I haven't had a chance to rest or step beyond the fast pace of a day. When I've taken a walk at lunch, paused to pray, or given myself space in a day or a week to cease, I am better able to demonstrate my love for him through my words and actions. The same goes for my son. When he does not have time to rest, he gets moody and whiny, and has emotional meltdowns. When he does rest, he is better able to cope with the huge demands placed on his little body and growing mind.

The peaceful act of sabbath is vital to our sacred balance because it holds the stillpoint between our steadiness and movement, doing and being, relationships with others and with ourselves. I invite you now into an examination of how you can make sabbath an intentional part of your rhythm. How might your work, whatever it may be, be rooted in the work of love and wisdom of peace?

Questions for Reflection

- Do you regularly set aside time to rest?
- If not, why? How could you shift your priorities to make space for rest and renewal? If so, how and when do you do it? What types of sabbath-keeping work well for you?
- What will make your sabbath holy?
- What does it mean to you to be a human being and a human doing?
- How do you practice nonviolence through self-care?

Wellness Practice: Create Sabbath Time

Keeping sabbath is a wellness practice in and of itself. It takes effort and intention to dedicate time for letting go of productivity. So often we wear our busyness as a badge of honor; letting go of our to-dos can feel like a giant and perhaps dangerous waste of time. We fear we will get hopelessly behind on our work. The truth is, the work will always be there. Sabbath helps us approach the work of life from a place of nourishment and trust rather than depletion and anxiety.

Take a look at your calendar and commitments for the week ahead. Where can you find time—an hour, an evening, a day—to put aside work?

What activities, or lack thereof, would you like to include in your sabbath? Worship, asana, walking, reading, couch-sitting, outings with family and friends? Whom would you like to share your sabbath with?

Notice whether there are already rhythms of rest in your schedule. What activities help you move into a space of intentional sabbath? Do you clean your house so you can rest in its freshness? Buy groceries and enjoy cooking or baking? Or do you put all that aside and do nothing?

When you've determined the time for your sabbath, tell a friend or loved one about it. Giving voice to your commitment to rest will help you stay accountable. You might even invite your friends and family to join you in a sabbath practice.

Continue to spend time each week with your calendar—either in your head, on the computer, or on paper—and commit to regular periods of otherwise unscheduled time to rest and refresh.

Meditation: Fallow Ground

Fallow ground is land that has been plowed and left unseeded for a season or more in order to restore its fertility. The practice of sabbath, with its intentional focus on spiritual connection and rest, plows out the weeds and overgrown crops in our lives and gives us time to breathe, reset, and prepare for the next phase of growth. In the following meditation we cultivate a fallowness of mind and heart in support of sabbath practice.

Take a comfortable seat on the floor, a chair, or a meditation cushion. Slowly close your eyes and turn your attention to your breath. Welcome in a few deep inhales and complete exhales, clearing the way for your body and mind to settle.

As your breath moves in a slow and comfortable rhythm, begin to visualize an open field. Notice the sky above and the trees on the borders of the land. Walk out into the field and feel the overgrowth of crops that have already born fruit, weeds that populate the spaces between rows of plantings. Each of these represent an aspect of your life or day whose time has passed.

Start to plow the field in your imagination, tilling the soil and cutting out the roots of the crops and other growth. The work is easy, for the soil is ready to be overturned. As you plow, the withered vegetation falls to the ground and mixes in the warm earth. It is not abandoned or destroyed. It is surrendered to the earth to decompose and restore nutrients.

When the field is fully plowed, put away your tools and rest. Breathe in the image of the tilled, empty land warmed by the sun, watered by rain, walked upon by foxes, and pecked at by birds. The land rests in communion with the beings and cycles of the natural world.

This open land is a part of you. Watch the earth breathe. Watch as it grows thankful for the gift of time to restore and renew instead of to produce. Stay with this image for some time.

When you are ready, slowly deepen your breath and open your eyes. Give thanks for this fallow, sabbath rest.

Asana Practice: Restorative Poses

A restorative yoga practice is similar to yin in that it involves long holds. It differs, however, in its use of props to reduce any strain on the body. Restorative yoga makes the poses passive and allows for even longer holds of five or ten or sometimes even twenty minutes. If you've ever used pillows to prop yourself up in bed to rest, you've done a form of restorative yoga.

Like yin, restorative asanas stimulate a wellspring of rejuvenation as they soothe the nervous system, promote a clear flow of prana, and ease the mind. There is no force or effort in restorative yoga but simply rest. As such, these postures are a perfect sabbath companion.

The asanas below can be done in sequence or on their own as a stand-alone practice.

Supported Supta Baddha Konasana: Supported Reclining Bound Angle Pose

This is one of the most potent restorative asanas because it opens the chest, abdomen, and hips without the effort required in other backbends. It counteracts habitual slouching and encourages trust in the support of Grace.

Setup takes a bit of effort, but once it is done, you can fully relax. For this asana, you will need a bolster or several folded blankets with optional blocks. The idea is to create a firm base, about 2½ feet long and 1 to 1¼ feet wide, upon which you can recline.

Once you have your stack ready, sit close to the edge and lie back. Your sitting bones will be on the floor and the base of the bolster or blankets near your lower back. Adjust your positioning so there is no strain. Gently lift and roll your shoulders under so that your shoulder blades are broad on the bolster and your chest expands. Let your arms hang down to the floor. This creates a slight back-bending action to stimulate the heart center.

Bring your feet together and let your knees lower out to the side. If there is a sensation of strain or pulling in your groin, elevate your knees with blocks or blankets.

Play around with the height of your blankets or bolster. If there is too much strain in your lower back, reduce the height to perhaps one blanket. For neck support, you may also place a small towel under your head. If you are unable to come to a place of ease, avoid this pose for the time being and move on to the next posture.

Once you find a comfortable position, close your eyes and rest. Breathe deep into your belly to help soften your body and mind. Stay here for five to twenty minutes.

To come out of the pose, slowly open your eyes and bring your knees together. Gently roll off the bolster or blankets and then rest on your side before pressing up to a comfortable seat.

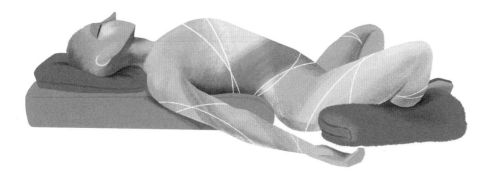

Viparita Karni: Legs Up the Wall Pose

Legs Up the Wall is a passive inversion. Inversions such as Head Stand and Shoulder Stand are among the more advanced yoga poses. Inversions reduce swelling in the legs and promote vitality by increasing blood flow to the brain, stimulating the pineal and thyroid glands, lowering blood pressure, and elevating mood. But it takes time to build the strength, mobility, and body awareness necessary to perform these asanas without injury. Legs Up the Wall is a lovely alternative that offers many of the same benefits without the need for technical know-how.

To begin, find a comfortable space by a wall where there is enough room to extend your legs up and your arms out to the side. Sit on the floor with your legs parallel to the wall. Roll to the side and swing your legs up the wall. Adjust your distance from the wall so that your tailbone and buttocks are resting on the floor and there is no strain in your low back. If your chin lifts too far to the sky or there is strain in your neck, place a small, folded blanket under your head.

If you have strain behind your knees, sit a little further away from the wall so you can bend your knees and rest your feet or heels on the wall.

Stretch your arms out to the side. Welcome a few long, slow breaths deep into your soft belly. Observe the sensation of the blood and fluid in your legs flowing downward to the basin of your pelvis. Close your eyes and breathe. Be here for five to ten minutes.

When you are ready, open your eyes and bend your knees to your chest before rolling to the side. Pause and come up to a comfortable seat.

Savasana: Corpse Pose

Corpse Pose is restorative as is, but it can be made even more so by placing a rolled blanket under the knees or a folded blanket across the thighs and pelvis. You may also place low support, such as a folded dish towel or hand towel, under your head.

To prepare, place your chosen props under or on your body and then lie down. Remain supine and stretch your arms and legs out. Let your feet relax out to the side. Gently lift your chest and roll your shoulders under so your shoulder blades are broad and your front body is expansive. Turn your palms up. Close your eyes.

Bring your awareness in toward the cavern of space in your torso. Allow it to expand as you move into the darkness of rest. Perhaps imagine roots growing from your spine, arms, and legs into the earth, where you can tap into the nourishment of the Ground of Being. Welcome yourself to this place of love. Breathe and rest here for five to seven minutes.

When you are ready, invite small movements back to your body and then roll to one side. Pause for a breath or two, then press up to a comfortable seat. Bring your hands together in front of your heart and offer thanks for your practice, for the support of friends and family who make this possible, and to the God of your understanding who walks with you on the path of sacred balance.

ACKNOWLEDGMENTS

While the physical act of writing is solitary, the process is done in community. I wish to take a small moment to thank everyone who contributed to the creation of this book and the fulfillment of this dream.

To Mom and Dad, who love and support me unconditionally. You gave and give me the space to grow, to question, and to ponder, and held me through many, many dark nights. I could not do this without you. And to my brother, Adam, who helps me shape ideas and pushes me to be a better writer. To Doug for tools, and Jeff, Peggy, and Mark for last-minute childcare.

An abundance of thanks to Christine Valters Paintner, who has taught me so much about the Benedictine path, and whose generosity of spirit connected me to Lil Copan at Broadleaf Books. Lil saw the seeds of this book and advocated to give it life. Thank you, Lil!

To Valerie Weaver-Zercher, my wonderful editor at Broadleaf, who asks all the right questions and helped shape and clarify this book. Your keen insight and kindness are invaluable. Thanks to Katherine Willis Pershey for feedback on the early draft. And to Alyssa Lochner, Claire Vanden Branden, and the Broadleaf Books team for putting so much effort into this work. I'm thrilled to work with you! Special thanks to Gisela Bohórquez for the lovely illustrations.

To Melissa Grantham, my soul sister, who always reminds me to breathe. Thank you to my cheerleading squad: Abby, Alice, Ashley, Callie, Katey, Michelette, Lori, and Stephanie, for your friendship and love. Deep gratitude to Mike Hubbell, my "boss" and friend who, upon hearing about this project said, "How can I support you in this?" and then meant it. And to everyone at the Y who joined him in giving me space to write.

Gratitude to the parish family of St. Paul's Episcopal, who live hospitality and care for me whether I'm active and serving or just hanging around the margins.

Abiding thanks to my teachers, especially Lila Rasa, who taught me yoga; Bill Mahony, who models kindness and love; and Cate Stillman, for lessons in Ayurveda. With gratitude for my students and colleagues who embarked upon this journey as we explored, and continue to explore, the dialogue between Benedictine spirituality and yoga.

To Ellis Peters for writing the Chronicles of Brother Cadfael, which introduced me to Benedictine life and provided refuge and hope during depression.

And finally, to Cole, who is too young to understand what this means, yet played patiently with Amma when I needed extra time to write. You are the love of my life.

RESOURCES FOR FURTHER STUDY

Ayurveda

Books

Ballentine, Rudolph. *Radical Healing: Integrating the World's Great Therapeutic Traditions to Create a New Transformative Medicine*. Honesdale, PA: Himalayan Institute, 2011.

Bhattacharya, Bhaswati. *Everyday Ayurveda: Daily Habits That Can Change Your Life*. New York: Penguin Random House, 2014.

Douillard, John. *Perfect Health for Kids: Ten Ayurvedic Health Secrets Every Parent Must Know*. Berkeley, CA: North Atlantic Books, 2004.

Stillman, Cate. *Body Thrive: Uplevel Your Body and Your Life with 10 Habits from Ayurveda and Yoga*. Boulder, CO: Sounds True, 2019.

Yarema, Thomas, Daniel Rhoda, and Johnny Brannigan. *Eat-Taste-Heal: An Ayurvedic Cookbook for Modern Living*. Kapa'a, HI: Five Elements, 2006.

Websites

www.Ayurveda.com

www.LifeSpa.com

www.YogaHealer.com

Benedictine Life

Books

Chittister, Joan. *The Rule of St. Benedict: A Spirituality for the 21st Century*. New York: Crossroad, 2010.

— — —. *Wisdom Distilled from the Daily: Living the Rule of St. Benedict Today*. New York: HarperOne, 2009.

de Waal, Esther. *Seeking God: The Way of St. Benedict*. Collegeville, MN: Liturgical Press, 2001.

Derkse, Wil, and Martin Kessler. *The Rule of Benedict for Beginners: Spirituality for Daily Life*. Collegeville, MN: Liturgical Press, 2003.

McQuiston II, John, and Phyllis Tickle. *Always We Begin Again: The Benedictine Way of Living*. New York: Morehouse, 2011.

Norris, Kathleen. *The Cloister Walk*. New York: Riverhead Books, 1996.

Paintner, Christine Valters. *The Artist's Rule: Nurturing Your Creative Soul with Monastic Wisdom*. Notre Dame, IN: Sorin Books, 2011.

— — —. *Lectio Divina — The Sacred Art: Transforming Words and Images into Heart-Centered Prayer*. Nashville, TN: SkyLight Paths, 2011.

Tomaine, Jane. *St. Benedict's Toolbox: The Nuts and Bolts of Everyday Benedictine Living*. New York: Morehouse, 2015.

Websites

www.AbbeyoftheArts.com

www.JoanChittister.org

www.MonasteriesoftheHeart.org

Yoga

Books

Brower, Elena, and Erica Jago. *Art of Attention: A Yoga Practice Workbook for Movement as Meditation*. Boulder, CO: Sounds True, 2016.

Farhi, Donna. *Bringing Yoga to Life: The Everyday Practice of Enlightened Living*. New York: HarperCollins, 2003.

Desikachar, T. K. V. *The Heart of Yoga: Developing a Personal Practice*. Rochester, VT: Inner Traditions, 1999.

Gates, Rolf, and Katrina Kenison. *Meditations from the Mat: Daily Reflections on the Path of Yoga*. New York: Anchor, 2002.

Iyengar, B. K. S. *Light on Yoga: The Bible of Modern Yoga*. New York: Schocken, 1995.

———. *Light on the Yoga Sūtras of Patañjali*. New York: Thorsons, 2002.

———. *The Tree of Yoga*. Boulder, CO: Shambhala, 2002.

Lasater, Judith Hanson. *Relax and Renew: Restful Yoga for Stressful Times*. Boulder, CO: Rodmell, 2005.

Mahony, William K. *Exquisite Love: Reflections on the Spiritual Life Based on Nārada's Bhakti Sūtras*. Vancouver, BC: Sarvabhava, 2014.

GLOSSARY

Author's Note: The terminology below, used in the pages of this book, comes from Sanskrit and from Latin. The definitions come from my studies and understanding of the concepts and are not necessarily strict linguistic or literal translations of each word.

abhyanga: Oil massage.

abhyasa: Steady effort over time.

ahimsa: Non-harming, or nonviolence; an unwillingness to do harm.

asana: A physical posture of yoga. A steady, comfortable seat; to sit comfortably and well. One of the eight limbs of yoga.

asteya: Non-stealing.

aparigraha: Non-clinging; letting go.

Ayurveda: The science of life. The traditional, holistic health and wellness modality of India.

brahmacharya: Walking with God; moderation, temperance.

conversatio morum: Conversion of life. The Benedictine vow of commitment to growth and daily improvement.

daya: An active expression of compassion; a generosity of spirit.

dharana: Concentration. One of the eight limbs of yoga.

dhyana: Meditation or contemplation. One of the eight limbs of yoga.

dina charya: Daily rhythms.

dosha: A category of energy made up of the interplay between qualities of space, air, earth, fire, and water. Describes patterns seen in the body, mind, and spirit; in the cycles of the day; and in the seasons of the year.

garshana: Dry brushing of skin.

hatha: A spiritual yoga practice using primarily asana and pranayama—movement and breath—as the main tools for balancing opposites. Can mean "willful"; refers to the sun and moon.

ishvara pranidhana: Surrender to God.

karuna: Compassion.

kapha: The dosha of earth and water.

lectio divina: Sacred reading.

namaste: "I bow to you." A greeting and an attitude that recognize the Divine Consciousness. Christians might interpret this to mean a recognition of the indwelling Christ in all of us.

nadi: Channel of energy.

niyamas: Observances for self-discipline and spiritual study.

oboedire: To listen, to hear; root of "obedience"; one of the vows taken by Benedictine monks and oblates.

pitta: The dosha of fire and water.

prana: Life force; life energy; breath.

pranayama: Techniques and practices for breath expansion and restraint.

pratyahara: Withdrawal of the senses.

rajas: Energy of fire and movement.

ritu charya: Seasonal rhythms.

shaucha: Purity; cleanliness outside and in.

samadhi: State of ecstasy, or merging with the highest form of the Self. One of the eight limbs of yoga.

santosha: Contentment.

sattva: Energy of clarity, equanimity, and balance.

satya: Truth; honesty.

spanda: Dynamic pulsation of life.

stabilitas: Stability; one of the vows taken by Benedictine monks and oblates.

sushumna nadi: Channel of Grace; central energetic channel in the body.

svadhyaya: Study of Self and scriptures.

tamas: Energy of heaviness and inertia.

tapas: Burning zeal in practice; desire to know more and willingness to grow.

vata: The dosha of space and air.

vinyasa: A generic term for a linked series of poses that flow from one to the next, in coordination with the breath and with little pause in between.

yamas: Moral and ethical guidelines for behavior.

yoga: A state of union; to unify and balance dynamic opposites.